YOGA FOR HEALTHY FEET

YOGA

FOR HEALTHY FEET

PRACTICE FROM THE GROUND UP

▼   ▼   ▼   ▼   ▼   ▼   ▼   ▼   ▼

Donald Moyer

SHAMBHALA   BOULDER, 2016

Shambhala Publications, Inc.
2129 13th Street
Boulder, Colorado 80302
www.shambhala.com

A Rodmell Press book

Printed in the United States of America

Shambhala Publications makes every effort to print on acid-free, recycled paper.

Shambhala Publications is distributed worldwide by Penguin Random House, Inc., and its subsidiaries.

Editors: Holly Hammond, Linda Cogozzo
Design: Gopa & Ted2, Inc.
Cover and Model Photo: Brian McDonnell
Author Photo: David Martinez Studio
Asana Illustrations: Gopa Campbell
Anatomy Illustrations: Lauren Keswick
Asana Model: Ada Lusardi
Lithographer: Walsworth Print Group

Library of Congress Cataloging-in-Publication Data
Moyer, Donald, 1939–
Yoga for healthy feet: practice from the ground up / Donald Moyer.
p. cm. — (Rodmell press yoga shorts)
Includes index.
ISBN 9781930485372 (pbk.: alk. paper)
1. Yoga. I. Title.
RA781.67 .M69 2016
613.7'046—dc23

2017275997

Contents

▼ ▼ ▼ ▼ ▼ ▼ ▼ ▼ ▼ ▼ ▼

Acknowledgments 7

Introduction 9

PART 1: Anatomy and Alignment 15

PART 2: The Learning Poses 45

PART 3: Practice Sequences 103

About the Author 119

From the Publisher 121

Index 123

Acknowledgments

▼ ▼ ▼ ▼ ▼ ▼ ▼ ▼ ▼ ▼ ▼ ▼

I AM DEEPLY grateful to Ada Lusardi, Vicky Palmer, Barbara Papini, Jennifer Sadugor, Candace Satlak, Joseph Satlak, Shari Ser, and Sandy Zirulnik for reading my manuscript with such diligent care and offering such helpful suggestions.

Special thanks to Ada Lusardi for her patience and good humor in modeling for both the inside and cover of this book, and to Gopa Campbell for bringing the poses to life with her skillful yoga illustrations.

This book has benefited at every stage of its development from the vision and expertise of Linda Cogozzo, copublisher at Rodmell Press.

Finally, heartfelt thanks to my students of the past forty-plus years for encouraging me to grow and evolve as a teacher, and to my fellow teachers at The Yoga Room in Berkeley, CA, for their continuing support.

Introduction

▼ ▼ ▼ ▼ ▼ ▼ ▼ ▼ ▼ ▼ ▼

OUR FEET SERVE two basic functions. They must be flexible enough to allow the intricate movements required for walking, running, and otherwise adapting to a changing terrain, yet strong enough to support the entire body in an upright position.

When our feet are encased in shoes, we tend to lose our awareness of the inner workings of the feet, in particular, the fanlike action of the metatarsals and the special function of each individual toe. Instead, we treat the feet like monolithic blocks, inert and dull.

The practice of yoga, especially the standing poses, allows us the freedom to go barefoot and make direct contact with the ground beneath us. For me, there is nothing as revitalizing to my nervous system as standing in Mountain Pose on a hardwood floor. Even using a nonskid mat feels like a degree of separation.

The chief aim of this book is to help you develop a kinesthetic awareness of your feet by familiarizing you with some basic anatomical landmarks, exploring the use of props such as wedges, blocks, and straps, and finding the optimum balance between strength and flexibility in your practice with the feet.

How to Use This Book

Yoga for Healthy Feet is divided into three parts. Part 1: Anatomy and Alignment describes the most important anatomical features of the feet from a yogic perspective: the toes and metatarsals, the balls of the feet, the inner and outer arches, the tarsal bones of the mid-foot, and the heels and ankles (page 17). I also introduce two special trigger points I discovered in my practice that you will not find in *Gray's Anatomy*: the inner corner of the ball of big toe and the inner corner of the heel (page 34).

In reading part 1, you will become more aware of the uniqueness of your own feet—the shape and habitual placement of your feet, how your toes align with your metatarsals, whether you have high or low arches, whether or not your ankle joints are flexible.

Part 1 also gives an overview of some of the most common problems affecting the feet, such as curled or hammer toes, bunions, high arches, low and fallen arches, sprained ankles, foot cramps, and plantar fasciitis. It includes guidelines on how to manage or alleviate each of these conditions through the practice of yoga.

The main emphasis in part 1, however, is not on therapeutic techniques as such, but on bringing the bones, muscles, and joints of the feet into balance, and maintaining that balance as the feet respond to a variety of circumstances. For optimum health, the foot should be properly aligned in all three dimensions—the inner foot balancing the outer foot, the balls of the foot balancing the heel, the top of the foot balancing the sole.

Please take your time in reading part 1. A great deal of information is packed into this section, so you may need to read it more than once, or refer back to certain sections when questions arise in the future.

Part 2: The Learning Poses presents mainly standing poses, because they teach us the most about the feet in particular, about alignment in general, and about balance overall. In addition to the standing poses, part 2 includes some basic sitting poses that are especially challenging for the feet and ankles.

Practice the poses in part 2 in the order presented. You may need more than one practice session to cover all the poses in the sequence. Work slowly and carefully to develop your awareness. Paying attention can be quite arduous, so when you begin to feel tired or lose concentration, end with a long Relaxation Pose and continue with the sequence in your next practice session.

The description for each pose includes:

- the name of the pose in English and Sanskrit

- the special benefits of the pose as practised in this book

- cautions about practicing the pose

- recommended and optional props

- instructions for practicing the pose with emphasis on the feet

- Practice Notes giving further suggestions

Try the recommended props for each pose, and note which ones are effective for you. Some of the props should be used every time you practice a particular pose, some can be used occasionally, while others may not be at all suited for your particular body. For example, if your feet cramp whenever you practice Hero Pose, using a support under your ankles at all times is advisable. If your feet don't cramp, but the pose feels better when your ankles are supported, use the prop only occasionally, such as on days when you feel stiffer than usual. If the prop makes no discernible difference, or makes you feel worse, then dispense with it altogether. There is no point in using a prop unless it helps you feel better in the pose. Consider it a favorable sign when a prop relieves pain or discomfort, allows greater movement, improves strength and balance, creates space in the joints, makes breathing easier, releases tension, or just plain feels good.

The Practice Notes for each pose provide suggestions that are intended for more experienced students and teachers. If you are a beginning student and feel overwhelmed by too much information, skip over this section for the time being and return to it when you are more familiar with the poses.

Part 3: Practice Sequences opens with a number of questions frequently asked by beginners: What if I have an injury or other health issue? What if I'm pregnant? When can I eat? What should I wear? What props do I need? The remainder of part 3 consists of five practice sequences drawn from the poses in part 2. Each sequence begins with a short description of the purpose of the sequence and practice notes that relate to the sequence.

The poses in the sequence are listed in practice order. For each pose, the English name and recommended prop (if any) is given, followed by the page number where a description of the pose can be found, and finally a suggested length of time for holding each pose.

If you follow the timings suggested, the practice sequences should take about 30 minutes each. Work at the pace that feels right for you. You may want to hold the poses longer than specified, or you may want to hold them for shorter periods, or repeat some of the poses two or three times. Find the rhythm of practice that feels most nourishing for you.

The first sequence, Find Your Feet, is a general sequence that focuses on three of the principal images and instructions for the feet used in this book. This sequence is best practiced without the use of any props for your feet, except for a nonskid mat. Practice this sequence a number of times, until you feel you have understood and assimilated the cues for your feet without the distraction of props. Return to this sequence when you feel that your body needs reminders.

The other four sequences are more therapeutic—that is, they focus on the use of props to alleviate problems and imbalances of the feet and ankles, such as hammertoes, bunions, sprained ankles, and weak arches. Practice a therapeutic sequence when it addresses your particular need. If a therapeutic sequence feels beneficial to you, return to it in your home practice once a week, once every two weeks, or whenever it feels appropriate.

Cautions related to the feet, ankles, and knees are included in the pose descriptions in part 2. In addition, here are some general cautions that apply to the whole of your yoga practice:

- Consult with your doctor or health care professional before embarking on a yoga practice if you have a chronic health problem or unresolved injury that might affect your participation.

- Do not continue to practice if you feel feverish, dizzy, nauseous, or breathless.

- Come out of a pose immediately if you feel a sharp pain in any of your joints or spine. Eliminate the pose from your routine until you can seek the advice of an experienced yoga teacher.

Part 1

▼ ▼ ▼ ▼ ▼ ▼ ▼ ▼ ▼ ▼ ▼

Anatomy and Alignment

In ALIGNING AND BALANCING the body as a whole and the feet in particular, no pose is more important than Mountain Pose. In our yoga practice, we begin each standing pose from the strength and quiet of Mountain Pose and return to it after each pose as our resting place. In Mountain Pose, we learn how the placement and action of the feet affect the rest of the body—knees, pelvis, spine, shoulder girdle, neck, and head.

In developing awareness of your feet, it is helpful to consider each of the three planes or dimensions separately (Figure 1): the inner and outer foot (sagittal plane), the top and bottom (transverse plane), and the front and back (frontal plane). As you will discover, each of these planes governs a different aspect or realm of the body.

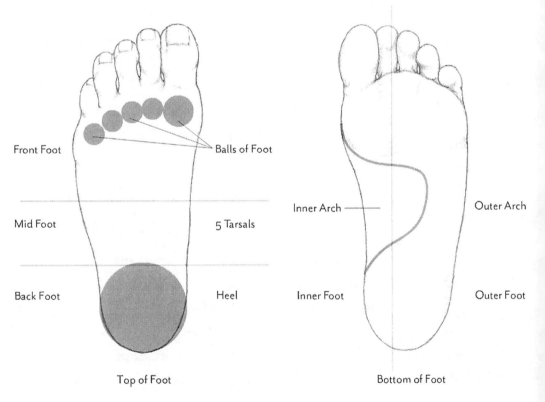

I. THE YOGA FOOT: TOP AND BOTTOM VIEWS

Inner and Outer Feet. How you stand on your inner and outer feet affects the rotation of your legs, the health of your knees, and ultimately the symmetry of your whole body.

If you stand habitually on your inner feet, your legs will rotate internally, putting pressure on your inner knees and leading ultimately to knock-knees. If you stand solely on your outer feet, your legs will rotate externally, putting strain on your outer knees and creating a tendency toward bowlegs.

If your right and left feet point in different directions, your knees and legs will reflect the unevenness, your pelvis may be torqued, and your whole torso will be asymmetrical. A minor imbalance in your feet can be magnified as it moves higher up the body.

Ideally, when you stand evenly on your inner and outer feet, your knees will point directly forward, with the heads of your thighbones centered in your hip sockets, neither rotating in nor rotating out, but in a neutral position that best supports the pelvis.

Top and Bottom. Working in the transverse plane, we coordinate the action of the bones of the top of the foot with the muscles of the sole of the foot. Here we are concerned with the effects of gravity, attempting to find a balance between the downward movement that brings a feeling of groundedness and the upward lift that brings lightness and ease.

Finding the balance between stability and lift depends to a great extent on the strength and resilience of the muscles of the arch. If the muscles and ligaments of the arch are too lax, they will not give proper support to the bones. If the muscles and ligaments of the arch are too tight, the bones will be forced upward and will not provide stability. In a well-balanced foot, the bones of the arch move down to meet the muscles of the arch, and the muscles of the arch lift up to support the bones.

Front and Back. Working in the frontal plane of the body, we divide our weight evenly between the balls of the feet and the heels. Balancing the front and the back of the foot in this way is essential for maintaining the natural curves of the spine.

When you stand habitually with your weight back on your heels, you tend to hyperextend (lock) your knees, tilt your pelvis forward, and overarch your lumbar spine. When you stand with your weight predominantly on the balls of your feet, you may slightly bend your knees, push your pelvis forward, and flatten your lumbar spine.

When your weight is divided evenly between the balls of your feet and your heels, your knees are firm but not locked, your pelvis balances lightly on the heads of your femurs, and your lumbar spine maintains its natural curve.

Feet Together or Feet Apart?

Students often ask, "In Mountain Pose, should my feet be together or apart? Which way is correct?"

Ultimately there is no single right way to practice a pose. Different ways of placing your feet in Mountain Pose bring different benefits. When you stand with your feet a few inches apart, your balance is more stable and you feel more grounded. Here your ankles are vertically aligned with your hip joints, emphasizing the strength of the legs.

When you stand in Mountain Pose with your feet together in the classical way, your inner thighs are vertically aligned with your spine. In this position, your inner thighs feel stronger and your spine more lifted.

How you choose to place your feet depends on your body type and your intention. If you have problems with balance or your arches are weak, you may benefit more from standing with your feet apart. If you want to focus on the lift of the spine, then stand with your feet together. In *Yoga for Healthy Feet*, I ask you to stand with your feet apart in Mountain Pose to emphasize stability and bring more awareness to your feet.

The Shape of Your Feet

Stand in Mountain Pose (page 52) with your feet a few inches apart, and look at the shape of your feet. Are they long and narrow, like a rectangle? Or wide in front but narrow at the heel, like a triangle? Or somewhere in between? The shape of your foot will tell you whether your feet are too tight, too loose, or firm and flexible (Figures 2A and 2B).

If your feet are long and narrow, the space between your metatarsals (the long bones of the feet) is often tight and restricted, limiting your ability to widen the balls of your feet and spread your toes. In this case, focus on widening your feet by rolling the first metatarsals toward the inner foot and the outer metatarsals toward the outer foot to create space between the balls of the feet. (The head of the first metatarsal at the base of the big toe is commonly defined as the ball of the foot, but I find it helpful to consider that each toe has a ball, as indicated in Figure 1.)

If the front of your foot is naturally broad, the balls of your feet are generally flexible. In this case, you don't need to spread your toes or widen your metatarsals any further. Focus instead on lengthening your metatarsals and keeping them aligned with your toes. If you continue to widen your already-wide front foot, you are more likely to develop bunions.

As a general rule, try to balance widening the foot and lengthening the foot. If your foot is narrow, pay more attention to widening the balls of the foot. If the front of your foot is wide, focus on lengthening the toes and metatarsals. If the shape of your foot falls somewhere in between, both lengthen and widen.

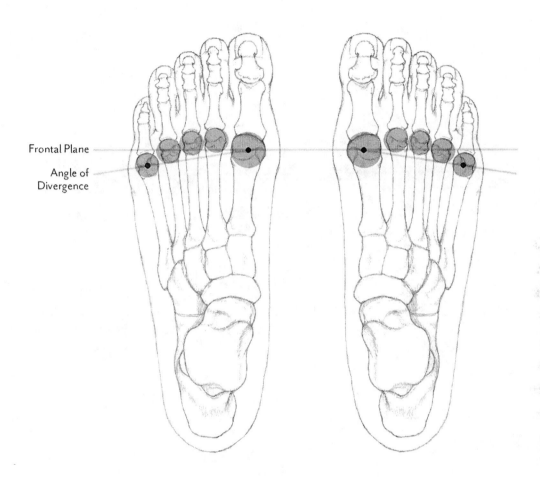

Frontal Plane

Angle of
Divergence

2A. THE SHAPE OF YOUR FOOT: LONG AND NARROW

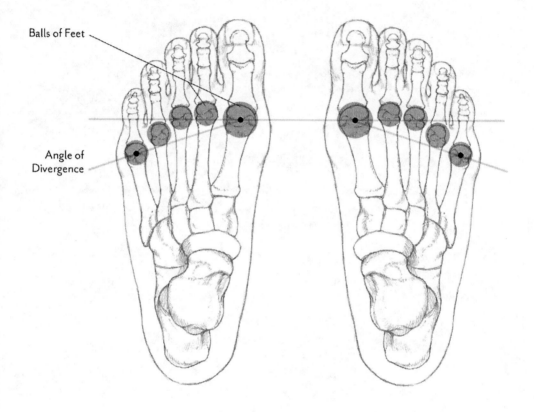

Balls of Feet

Angle of
Divergence

2B. THE SHAPE OF YOUR FOOT: SHORT AND WIDE

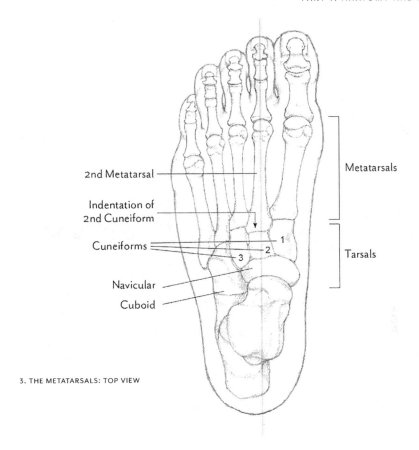

2nd Metatarsal

Indentation of
2nd Cuneiform

Cuneiforms

Navicular

Cuboid

Metatarsals

Tarsals

3. THE METATARSALS: TOP VIEW

The Metatarsals

The metatarsals are the long bones of the foot that connect the toes with the five tarsals that form the roof of the arch: the three cuneiforms, the navicular, and the cuboid (Figure 3).

Observe in Figure 3 how the first three metatarsals are joined to the three cuneiform bones at the top of the foot. Notice how the second cuneiform is set a little farther back than the first and third cuneiforms. The second metatarsal fits snugly into this indentation and is held in place laterally by the adjacent cuneiforms. The first metatarsal is free to roll toward the inner foot, and the outer metatarsals to roll toward the outer foot, but the lateral movement of the second metatarsal is restricted.

The second metatarsal moves up and down like a lever or drawbridge but does not revolve to the left or the right. Given its relative stability, it serves as a fence or dividing line between the inner and outer foot. The second metatarsal thus functions as the median line of the foot, reminding us to balance the greater power of the first metatarsal and big toe with the united strength and mobility of the outer three metatarsals and toes.

Aligning the Feet

In symmetrical standing poses such as Mountain Pose, Toe-Holding Pose, Chair Pose, Standing Forward Bend, Wide-Leg Standing Forward Bend, and Downward-Facing Dog Pose, align your feet so that the second metatarsals are parallel to each other and the second toes point directly forward (Figure 4). Roll your outer metatarsals toward your outer foot and your first metatarsals toward your inner foot, so that your inner and outer arches are evenly lifted.

There may be special circumstances in practicing a symmetrical standing pose where it is beneficial to turn your feet in or out, instead of pointing them directly forward. In Standing Forward Bend, for instance, allowing the feet to turn in encourages internal rotation of the thighs and can relieve sciatic pain that results from a tight piriformis muscle. On the other hand, allowing the feet to turn out in a squatting position can relieve strain on the knees and improve balance.

In asymmetrical standing poses such as Extended Triangle Pose, Extended Side-Angle Pose, Warrior II Pose, and Half Moon Pose, your feet are aligned separately. When practicing side-bending poses to the right, turn your right foot out so that the second metatarsal is parallel to the long edge of your mat. When placing your left foot, draw an imaginary line from the center of the ball of the big toe to the center

MAT

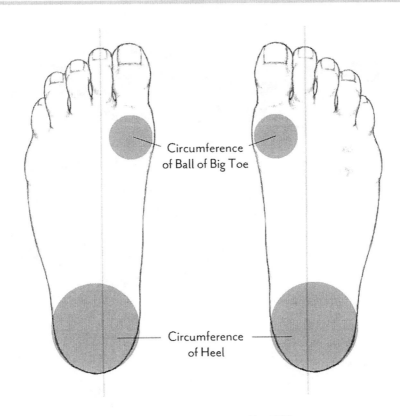

Circumference
of Ball of Big Toe

Circumference
of Heel

4. ALIGNING THE FEET IN SYMMETRICAL POSES

of the ball of the little toe. Then turn the foot in so that this line is parallel to the long edge of your mat. Aligning the back foot in this way gives you more leverage in firming and broadening the balls of the foot (Figures 5A and 5B).

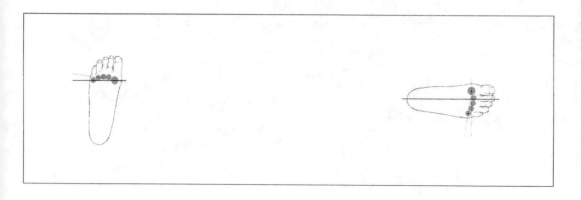

5A. ALIGNING THE FEET IN ASYMMETRICAL POSES: LONG AND NARROW

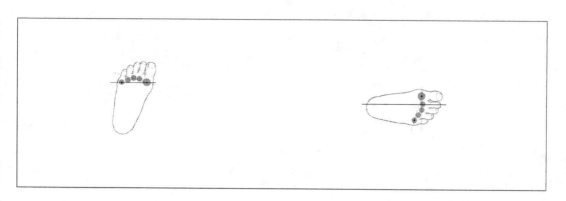

5B. ALIGNING THE FEET IN ASYMMETRICAL POSES: SHORT AND WIDE

Note that people with triangular-shaped feet, where the balls of the feet slant away from the frontal plane of the body at a significant angle, will need to turn the left foot in at a greater angle than those with long rectangular feet, where the balls of the feet are more in line with the frontal plane.

The Toes

In Mountain Pose, we begin by lengthening the toes and widening the metatarsals to establish the overall strength and balance of the feet. Next we align the toes with the metatarsals, so that each toe points in the same direction as its corresponding metatarsal, by lengthening the inner and outer edges of the toes evenly. If the inner edge lengthens more than the outer edge, the toe will veer toward the outer foot. If the outer edge lengthens more than the inner edge, the toe will veer toward the inner foot.

We should also consider the alignment of the segments within the toes themselves. The big toe has two segments: the tip of the toe (the distal or farthest segment) and the neck of the toe (the proximal or nearest segment). The other four toes each have three segments: the distal segment, known as the tip of the toe, the middle segment, and the proximal segment, referred to as the neck of the toe. In a healthy foot, the toes do not bend or curl but are relatively straight.

Mallet, Hammer, and Claw Toes. When the intrinsic muscles that flex or extend the toes are habitually overworked, or when the front of the foot is habitually compressed by ill-fitting shoes, the shape of the toes can be distorted in different ways, resulting in mallet toes, hammertoes, and claw toes (Figure 6).

In a mallet toe, the tip of the toe curls down and presses into the floor. You can simulate mallet toes by standing in Mountain Pose and gripping the floor with the tips of your toes. This action strengthens the tip of the toe but leaves the neck of the toe weak and foreshortened.

In a hammertoe, the neck of the toe lifts away from the floor and the toe itself curls. To simulate hammertoes, stand in Mountain Pose and pull your toes toward your metatarsals. As your toes lift away from the floor, notice how the tendons at the top of the foot stand out in sharp ridges. (If these ridges do not disappear when your toes are at rest, it indicates chronic tension and overwork in the top of the foot. In a well-balanced foot, the surface of the top of the foot is broad and smooth.)

In a claw toe, the tip of the toe presses down and the neck of the toe is lifted up—a combination of mallet toe and hammertoe.

If you have mallet, hammer, or claw toes, the most effective way to straighten your toes is by lengthening the neck of the toe away from the metatarsal. You may find it helpful to place a wedge under your toes, as described for Chair Pose (page 61). The wedge lifts the tip of the toes higher than the neck of the toes and allows you to lengthen the toes without gripping. The wedge is used in a number

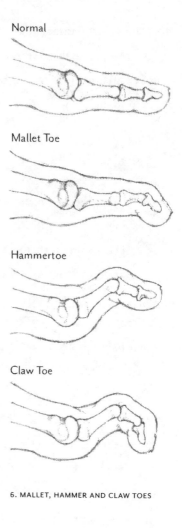

Normal

Mallet Toe

Hammertoe

Claw Toe

6. MALLET, HAMMER AND CLAW TOES

of poses in Practice Sequence 2: Strengthen Your Toes (page 110). This sequence is intended primarily for those with curled or hammer toes, but it will help to maintain the strength and integrity of your toes even if they are straight.

Toe-Straightening Exercise. Here is a simple toe-straightening exercise you can do while watching the evening news. Sit on a block or bolster with your right foot flat on the floor, and cross your left leg so that your left foot rests on the floor behind your right foot. Begin by adjusting the toes of your right foot. Place your right index finger lengthwise under the tip of your right second toe and your thumb on top of the neck of the toe. With your index finger, draw the fleshy pad from underneath the toe toward the very tip of the toe. At the same time, press gently with your thumb and lengthen the neck of the toe. Hold for a few seconds with the toe elongated. Then repeat for the third, fourth, and fifth toes.

To adjust your big toe, place fingers 2 through 5 under the corresponding toes of your right foot, and press your right thumb on the neck of the big toe. With your fingers, lift and lengthen toes 2 through 5. With your thumb, roll the neck of your big toe toward your inner foot and press down gently. When you have adjusted all the toes of the right foot, reverse your sitting position and adjust the toes of the left foot.

In this exercise, notice how each toe needs a slightly different adjustment. Some toes need to be turned as well as lengthened. For others, the pad at the tip of the toe needs to be more evenly rounded. You may find a toe that no longer fully straightens because one of the joints is locked in a bent position. Encourage this toe to lengthen as much as it can with the help of your fingers.

Big Toe Bunions

A bunion, or enlargement of the ball of the big toe, develops from the misalignment of the big toe and the first metatarsal. Especially when the front of the foot is wide and overly flexible, the ball of the big toe (in anatomical terms, the head of the first metatarsal) rolls toward the inner foot but the big toe turns toward the outer foot, that is, toward the second toe. Initially, the ball of the big toe is not compromised, but as the angle of divergence increases, the big toe gradually loses its strength, and the ball of the big toe becomes enlarged and often inflamed (Figure 7).

You can estimate the angle of divergence by measuring the intersection of the longitudinal axis (median line) of the first metatarsal with the longitudinal axis of the big toe. If the two axes are continuous, the big toe and first metatarsal are well aligned.

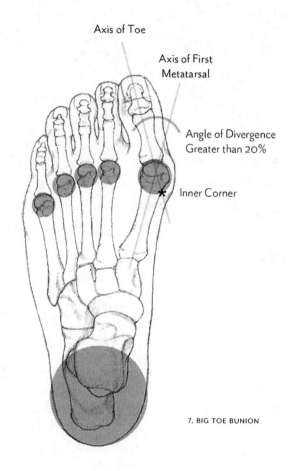

Axis of Toe

Axis of First
Metatarsal

Angle of Divergence
Greater than 20%

Inner Corner

7. BIG TOE BUNION

If the angle of divergence is less than 20 degrees, it is still considered within normal range by health care professionals.

If the angle of divergence is greater than 20 degrees, take a minute to compare your big toe with the ball of your big toe. Does the ball of the big toe look enlarged and gnarly? Does the big toe seem weaker than the ball of the big toe? Does the big toe retract toward the ball or does it extend forward? (When the big toe is strong and healthy, it lengthens forward.)

The propensity to develop bunions is often hereditary, but wearing shoes that do not fit properly and certain habitual ways of working with your feet, such as gripping your toes, forcefully spreading your toes, or pressing down unevenly on the ball of the big toe, can be contributing factors.

Here are some suggestions for managing your bunions or incipient bunions:

- **Don't grip the tips of your toes.** When you grip the floor with the tips of your toes, your big toes are weakened and pulled toward your second toes. If you find yourself gripping, relax the tips of your toes by lifting them slightly, and lengthen the neck of the big toes.

- **Strengthen the inner corner of the ball of your big toe.** In my experience, the muscles and ligaments that support the inner corner of the ball of the big toe (Figure 7) become looser and weaker as the angle of divergence of the big toe increases. To bring the big toe and first metatarsal into better alignment, it is essential to strengthen the inner corner of the ball of your big toe. You can make the following adjustment in Standing Forward Bend (page 72) or Chair Pose (page 61), or in sitting poses such as Head-of-the-Knee Pose (page 88) or Bound Angle Pose (page 91).

  First place your index finger between your big toe and second toe, and slide the tip of your thumb underneath the inner corner of the ball of your big toe. With your index finger, draw your big toe toward your inner foot so that it aligns with your first metatarsal. At the same time, firm the inner corner of the ball of your big toe against your thumb, and lengthen the neck of your big toe from there.

- **Spread your weight evenly around the circumference of the ball of your big toe.** In the past, yoga teachers have instructed their students to "press down with the ball of the big toe" to stabilize the front foot in standing poses. The problem with this direction is that most students, especially those with incipient bunions, press down heavily but unevenly on the ball of the big toe, which inadvertently increases the angle of divergence between the big toe and first metatarsal.

I prefer to draw an imaginary circle around the ball of the big toe and distribute the weight lightly and evenly around the circumference. I find that working with this image brings my big toe into better alignment with my first metatarsal, and keeps my incipient bunion from developing any further (Figure 7).

Inner and Outer Arches

The longitudinal arch of the foot is divided into the inner arch and the outer arch. The inner arch supports the first three metatarsals of the inner foot. The outer arch supports the fourth and fifth metatarsals of the outer foot.

In symmetrical poses such as Mountain Pose, observe the balance between your inner and outer arches. If you stand primarily on the outer edges of your feet, your inner arches will lift but your outer arches will drop. If you stand predominantly on your inner feet, your outer arches will lift but your inner arches will drop. To balance your weight on the feet, always lift the inner and outer arches evenly.

In asymmetrical poses such as Extended Triangle Pose, the weight tends to fall on the outer foot of the front leg and the inner foot of the back leg. To balance the foot of the front leg, focus on lifting the outer arch more. To balance the foot of the back leg, focus on lifting the inner arch more. If you have fallen arches, you may find that the weight falls on your inner foot on both legs. In any case, check that the inner and outer arches of both feet are lifting evenly in asymmetrical poses.

High, Low, and Fallen Arches

Some people have naturally high arches and others have naturally low arches, but having low arches should not be confused with having fallen arches. It doesn't matter how near or far the arch is from the floor, so long as the muscles of the arch lift into the bones, and the bones of the arch press into the muscles. You can practice lifting the muscles of the arch while pressing down with the bones most effectively in Reclining Toe-Holding Pose with a strap (page 47).

High Arches. When you have high arches, the bones of the arch tend to pull away from the muscles, leaving the muscles of the arch somewhat contracted and foreshortened. In this case, focus on widening and lengthening your metatarsals so that they come in better contact with the muscles of the arch.

If you have high arches, you may experience some discomfort when sitting on the top of your feet, as in Hero Pose, either from your arches cramping or from the intense pressure on the top of your feet. If this happens to you, practice Hero Pose (page 84) with your ankles supported to take the weight off the top of your feet. (Those with flat feet and tight ankles may benefit from this as well.)

If you have very high arches, you may have difficulty with your balance in the standing poses, and you may be susceptible to spraining your ankles. If you feel unsteady in the standing poses or if you are recovering from a sprained ankle, practice the standing poses with the heel of your back foot at the base of a wall, as described for Extended Triangle Pose (page 58) and Practice Sequence 3: Stabilize Your Foot and Ankle (page 112). Using a wedge under your toes, as described for Warrior Pose II (page 63) and Practice Sequence 2: Strengthen Your Toes (page 110), may also be helpful.

Low Arches. If you have low arches, the muscles of the arch tend to be lax and drop away from the bones of the arch. In this case, focus on lifting and strengthening the muscles of the arch so that they give more support to the bones. You can learn the proper movement by practicing Reclining Toe-Holding Pose with a strap (page 47).

When strengthening the muscles of the arch, I find it helpful to firm and lift the two points at either end of the inner arch—the inner corner of the heel and the inner corner of the ball of the big toe (Figure 8). I think of these points as the ends of a rainbow. When I firm and lift these points into the bone, the whole span of the inner arch feels stable and grounded.

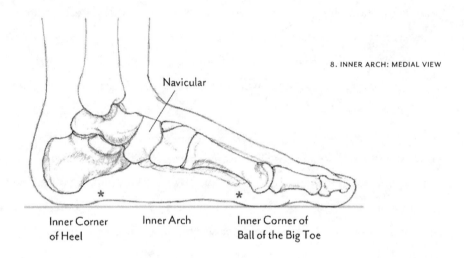

8. INNER ARCH: MEDIAL VIEW

Navicular

Inner Corner of Heel   Inner Arch   Inner Corner of Ball of the Big Toe

Fallen Arches. Let's return to the difference between low arches and fallen arches. With low arches, the muscles of the arch may be somewhat weak, but the bony structure of the foot is more or less intact. With fallen arches, however, there is a marked structural disorder: not only do the bones of the mid-foot appear radically displaced but the ankle joint loses its integrity and the inner anklebone collapses.

The tendency to drop the inner arch is most noticeable when coming into Downward-Facing Dog Pose. If you press your shinbones into the ankle joints in order to lower the heels, you will lose the lift of the arch and overwork your Achilles tendon.

To prevent the collapse of your arches in Downward-Facing Dog Pose (page 50), lift your shinbones away from your front ankle joints as you descend your heels.

If you have fallen arches, I recommend that you use a wedge or rolled mat under your heels in Downward-Facing Dog Pose (page 50) whenever you practice the pose. With support under your heels, you can focus on maintaining the lift of your shinbones by relaxing the front of your ankle joints, lengthening your lower calf muscles away from your Achilles tendons, and broadening your heels. This movement creates space in the ankle joints and allows the bones of the foot to realign.

The Five Tarsals: Bones of the Mid Foot

The mid foot consists of a group of five small bones collectively known as the five tarsals, which together form the roof of the arch. The three cuneiforms separate the first three metatarsals from the outer two metatarsals and create a split-level division between the inner and outer arch. The navicular acts as the keystone for the high vault of the inner arch, and the cuboid is the keystone for the lower vault of the outer arch (Figures 9A, 9B, and 9C).

Ideally the saddle-like area of the mid foot between the metatarsals and the front ankle should appear smooth and broad, with no bumps or protuberances disturbing the surface. However, if this area is tight and narrow, you may feel a bony protrusion known as a saddle bump in the region of the third cuneiform.

In my experience, when the tarsal bones of the mid foot are tight and narrow, the movement of the ankle joint is restricted, and when the movement of the ankle joint is restricted, the knee joint becomes more vulnerable, especially when practicing sitting poses such as Head-of-the-Knee Pose and Simple Seated Twist II. To free the front ankle and protect the knee, it is essential to keep the bones of the mid foot soft and broad.

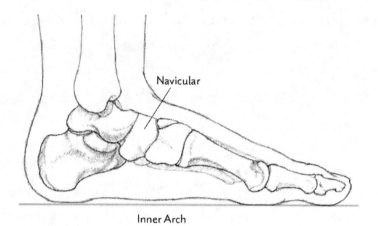

Inner Arch

9A. INNER ARCH: MEDIAL VIEW

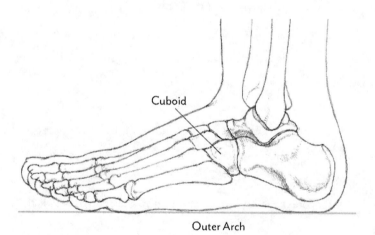

Outer Arch

9B. OUTER ARCH: LATERAL VIEW

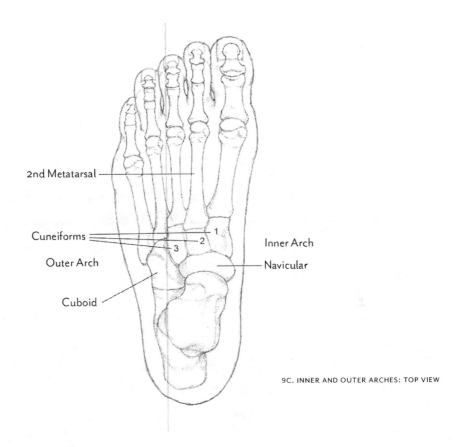

2nd Metatarsal

Cuneiforms

Outer Arch

Cuboid

Inner Arch

Navicular

9C. INNER AND OUTER ARCHES: TOP VIEW

The Heels

The heel bone, or calcaneus, is the largest bone in the foot. The ligaments of the plantar fascia attach to the front edge of the heel bone, and the Achilles tendon attaches to the back edge, thus linking the sole of the foot with the back of the lower leg.

If you have difficulty keeping the heel of your back foot in contact with the floor in standing poses such as Warrior Pose I (page 77), lift your lower calf muscle away from the Achilles tendon and broaden your heel. Notice I suggest that you "broaden the heel," not "dig the heel" or "grind the heel." When you dig or grind the heel into the floor, you jam the shinbone into the ankle joint and collapse your inner arch.

The fleshy pad of the heel should act like a shock absorber to protect the heel bone from the trauma of impact. So when you stand in Mountain Pose, broaden your heels and let them feel thick and cushiony.

Circumference of the Heels. The most effective way I have found for preserving the cushion of the heels is this: Start in Mountain Pose by drawing an imaginary circle around the pads of your heels, and then distribute your weight evenly around the whole circumference (Figure 4).

When you have balanced the heels front and back, inner and outer, bring your awareness to your knees. Draw an imaginary circle around each knee joint, and balance your weight evenly around the circumference. Then align the circumference of your knees with the circumference of your heels. Feel how this adjustment strengthens your legs and feet.

Inner Corner of the Heel. In assessing the circumference of the heels, you may find that the inner corner of the heel is lax and needs strengthening. To activate the inner corner of the heel, practice Reclining Toe-Holding Pose, Standing Forward Bend, and Staff Pose all with a strap around the arches. Remember to place the strap at the front edge of the heel so that you can firm the inner corner of the heel against the strap (Figure 8).

Plantar Fasciitis

If you experience a nagging pain in your heel, you may have plantar fasciitis, an inflammation of the connective tissue where it inserts at the front edge of the heel bone. Plantar fasciitis is often brought on by vigorous activity such as running, or by an occupation such as teaching or sales that requires you to stand on your feet for prolonged periods of time. The ligament of the plantar fascia, which attaches to the front of the calcaneus (heel bone), is especially vulnerable to microscopic pulls and tears, which can eventually cause such acute discomfort that walking becomes unbearable.

For the relief of plantar fasciitis, give your feet a rest until the pain has subsided enough for you to walk without limping. Apply an ice pack to your heels for about twenty minutes three or four times a day to relieve the inflammation. Check with your doctor about using an anti-inflammatory medication such as ibuprofen (Advil or Motrin) or naproxen (Aleve), either in pill form or as a cream to rub into the tender area. Wear comfortable shoes that support your arches and provide a healthy cushion for your heels.

If you suffer from plantar fasciitis, most podiatrists recommend that you do not walk barefoot at any time. Despite this warning, I encourage you to practice yoga without shoes if at all possible, once the pain has diminished. To minimize any residual discomfort, use a thicker mat to provide more of a cushion for your feet. Try placing a wedge under your heels to release the strain on your Achilles tendon.

To alleviate plantar fasciitis in your yoga practice, you need first of all to lengthen your Achilles tendons and then to balance your inner and outer arches.

Lengthen the Achilles Tendons. The most effective relief from the pain of plantar fasciitis comes from lengthening the Achilles tendons. How does this work? In plantar fasciitis, the muscles of the arch and their connective tissue are tight and constricted. In order to release and lengthen the bottom of the foot, you need to increase your range of motion in dorsiflexion, that is, by bringing the tops of your feet and your shins closer together.

In your yoga practice, you can work on dorsiflexion in Reclining Toe-Holding Pose with a strap (page 47) by holding your leg steady and pulling your foot closer to your shin. I personally find that flexing the heel in this way creates tension at the front of my ankle joint and makes the tendons at the top of my foot protrude. For me, this adjustment creates more problems than it solves.

I prefer to work on dorsiflexion by stabilizing the feet and pressing the shins closer to the top of the feet, as in Chair Pose (page 61). This allows your Achilles tendons to release and lengthen without tensing the top of the foot. If you are subject to plantar fasciitis, I recommend that you return to Chair Pose for a few breaths after each standing pose. In Chair Pose, press the top of your shinbones forward, let your lower calf muscles release away from your Achilles tendons, and simultaneously relax any tension at the front of your ankle joints. As your Achilles tendons lengthen, you may feel the muscles of your arch soften and lengthen as well.

Balance the Inner and Outer Arches. If you have plantar fasciitis, focus on lifting your inner and outer arches evenly in all the standing poses, especially those included in Practice Sequence 1: Find Your Feet (page 108). An imbalance between your inner and outer arches will put additional stress on your plantar fascia ligaments.

Foot Cramps

A cramp is a sudden, involuntary contraction of a muscle, which is often unbearably painful. In response to a muscle cramp, you instinctively stop whatever you are doing and massage the agonized muscle until the fierce gripping subsides. The spasm usually lasts for only a few seconds but is very intense.

If you experience muscle cramps frequently, you may have a nutritional deficiency in magnesium, calcium, or vitamin D. Alternatively you may suffer from dehydration, or the cramping may be related to a chronic illness such as diabetes or Parkinson's disease. If you are concerned about your tendency to cramp, you should consult your medical doctor.

In a yoga class, the most common form of cramping in my experience is the cramping of the muscles of the arch in poses where the top of the foot presses against the floor, such as Hero Pose and Camel Pose. In these poses, especially if the person has high arches, there is undue pressure on the top of the foot, together with overworking of the ankle joint. (You can often tell that the ankle joint is jammed or overworked by looking at the skin at the back of the heel. If the skin is blanched and colorless, it indicates a lack of circulation.)

You can avoid cramping of the arches in these poses by placing a rolled facecloth between the floor and the front of your ankle joint, as described in Hero Pose with ankles supported (page 84). When the ankle joints are supported in this way, they are no longer forced beyond their normal range of motion, the pressure on the top of the feet is relieved, and circulation to the feet and ankles improved. The skin at the back of the heel is no longer blanched.

Sprained Ankle

A sprained ankle is caused by the sudden impact of turning or twisting your foot as you stumble or fall, damaging the ligaments that support the ankle joint by over-stretching or tearing them. Most often the weight rolls onto the outer foot, trauma-tizing the ligaments of the outer ankle, but occasionally it rolls onto the inner foot, injuring the inner ankle.

When you sprain an ankle, you usually feel the pain and swelling right away. When this happens, rest your foot and avoid weight bearing. Consult a health care professional to rule out the possibility that you have fractured or broken a bone. Apply an ice pack to your injured ankle for twenty minutes at a time, and repeat at intervals of two or three hours. Wrap your sprained ankle in an elastic bandage to help reduce swelling. Lie with your foot elevated above the level of your heart.

Take a break from your yoga practice until the pain and swelling of your sprained ankle have completely subsided. If you begin weight bearing too soon, you are likely to reinjure your ankle. When your sprained ankle is pain-free, gradually reintroduce the standing poses to your routine, but hold them for only a few seconds each. Practice the standing poses with the outer heel of your back foot pressing into the wall, as described for Extended Triangle Pose (page 58), to strengthen and support your ankle. Practice Sequence 3: Stabilize Your Foot and Ankle (page 112) once or twice a week until your ankle has fully recovered and no longer feels vulnerable.

The Ankle Joint

At the back of the foot, the talus bone sits directly above the calcaneus (heel bone) and supports the tibia and fibula (the bones of the lower leg) to form the ankle joint (Figure 10).

The mobility of the ankle joint makes possible the four basic movements of the foot: pronation, supination, plantar flexion, and dorsiflexion. Our goal in practicing yoga is to extend our range of motion in all four directions without overworking or stressing the ankle joint.

Pronation. In pronating the foot (turning the top of the foot toward the inner foot), keep your inner anklebone lifted to avoid collapsing your inner arch, especially if you have low or weak arches.

To strengthen your feet in pronation, practice Standing Forward Bend with a strap around your arches (page 72). Firm the muscles of your arch against the strap, turn

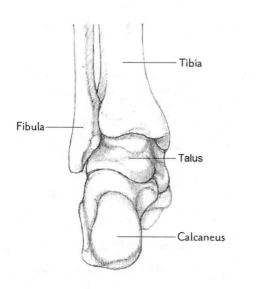
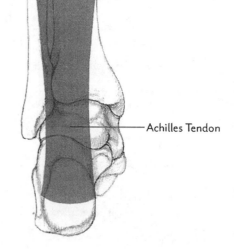

10. HEEL AND ANKLE JOINT: POSTERIOR VIEW

your first metatarsals in, and at the same time lift your inner anklebones away from the inner corners of your heels.

Supination. In supination (turning the top of the foot toward the outer foot), we want to avoid sickling the foot, which comes by overstretching the ligaments of the outer ankle joint and compressing the inner ankle joint. Sickling occurs most frequently in sitting poses such as Head-of-the-Knee Pose, Bound Angle Pose, and Simple Seated Twist II. In these poses, you can restore the ankle joint to a more neutral position by supporting the outer ankle with a rolled facecloth or other lift.

Sickling is also implicated in Wide-Leg Standing Forward Bend when you feel a burning sensation on the skin of your outer calf. In this case, roll your outer metatarsals toward your outer feet and your first metatarsals toward your inner feet to balance the inner and outer feet. If this doesn't relieve the burning sensation, try Wide-Leg Standing Forward Bend with your feet on wedges (page 70) to reduce the angle of supination.

To strengthen the feet in a supinated position, I recommend Standing Forward Bend with your feet on wedges (page 66). When I practice this variation immediately before a balancing pose such as Tree Pose or Half Moon Pose, I find that my balance improves.

Plantar Flexion. In plantar flexion, or pointing the foot, we want to open the front of the ankle joint without gripping the Achilles tendon or jamming the back of the ankle joint. You can practice this movement most effectively in Reclining Toe-Holding Pose with a strap around the arch of the raised leg (page 47) by activating the muscles of the arch as you lengthen your metatarsals toward the toes.

Plantar flexion can be problematic in poses such as Hero Pose, where the top of the foot presses against the floor. If you experience cramping or discomfort in your feet in this pose, you may be overworking your ankle joints. When this occurs, practice Hero Pose with your ankles supported (page 84) to ease the strain on your ankle joints by bringing them to a more neutral position.

Dorsiflexion. In dorsiflexion, or flexing the heel, we want to open the back of the ankle joint without gripping or hardening the front of the ankle joint. You can increase your range of motion in dorsiflexion most easily in Chair Pose (page 61), by relaxing the front of the ankle joint as you lengthen your Achilles tendon.

I avoid flexing the heels in sitting poses such as Staff Pose and Head-of-the-Knee Pose because I find that dorsiflexion in these poses overworks the tendons at the top of the foot, flattens the inner arches, and stresses the hamstrings. I prefer to use a strap around the arches, as described for Staff Pose (page 86), to stabilize the heel, lengthen the metatarsals, and thus maintain a neutral position of the ankle joint.

Part 2

▼ ▼ ▼ ▼ ▼ ▼ ▼ ▼ ▼ ▼ ▼

The Learning Poses

Reclining Toe-Holding Pose

SUPTA PADANGUSTHASANA

▼ ▼ ▼ ▼ ▼ ▼ ▼ ▼ ▼ ▼

strengthens the muscles of the arch ※ balances the inner and outer foot
※ recommended for those with low or fallen arches, but beneficial for all

Props: 1 nonskid mat ※ 1 strap

Optional Props: 1 blanket ※ 1 block, bolster, or wall

Reclining Toe-Holding Pose is practiced here with a strap around the foot of the raised leg (Figures 11 and 11A).

Lie on your back on a nonskid mat with your legs extended. (If you feel any strain in your neck, place a folded blanket under your head and neck.) Bend your right knee into the chest, and place a strap around the arch of your right foot so that the strap

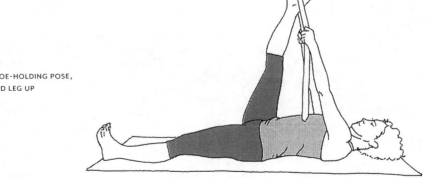

11. RECLINING TOE-HOLDING POSE,
WITH STRAP AND LEG UP

presses against the front edge of your heel. Then straighten your right leg, and hold the strap in both hands with your arms fully extended.

With Leg Up. With your right leg raised, firm the inner corner of your right heel, and press your first metatarsal into the strap. Relax the bones at the top of your right foot, and lengthen your metatarsals toward the toes so that your toes point toward the ceiling. With your left leg extended, firm the inner corner of your left heel, and widen the metatarsals of your left foot.

Remain in this position for about a minute. Check that the inner and outer arches of your right foot are lifted evenly. When you are ready, practice the next variation.

With Leg to Side. With your right leg raised, take hold of both ends of the strap with your right hand. Check that the strap is around the back of the arch, just in front of the heel. Place your left hand on your left hipbone with your elbow bent. With an inhalation, firm the inner corner of your right heel, and press your first metatarsal against the strap. With an exhalation, lengthen the metatarsals of your right foot as you lower your right leg out to the side. As your right leg descends, relax your lower abdomen but let your upper abdomen turn toward the left. (If your leg doesn't reach the floor, use a block, bolster, or wall to support the outer leg.)

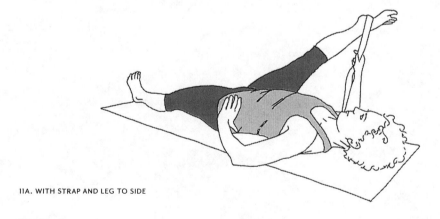

11A. WITH STRAP AND LEG TO SIDE

Remain in this position for about a minute. With your right leg out to the side, relax the bones at the top of your right foot, and press the first metatarsal against the strap. With your left leg extended, firm the inner corner of your left heel, and widen the metatarsals of your left foot.

To come out of the pose, raise your right leg away from the floor with an inhalation, and lower it to the floor with the exhalation. Then repeat the pose and variation with the left leg raised.

Practice Notes. Use the strap around the arch of the foot even if you are flexible enough to take hold of the big toe. The pressure of your foot against the strap helps to activate and strengthen the muscles of the arch.

Note that a wide strap is more effective for this pose than a narrow strap. If you are using a narrow strap (1 inch wide), fold the strap in half to double it. Place one strand at the front edge of the heel and the other strand alongside it across the center of the arch.

INVERTED POSE

Downward-Facing Dog Pose

ADHO MUKHA SVANASANA

▼ ▼ ▼ ▼ ▼ ▼ ▼ ▼ ▼ ▼ ▼

reduces strain of the Achilles tendon ▪ creates space in the ankle joints
▪ recommended if your heels do not reach the floor,
or if you have fallen arches or plantar fasciitis

Props: 1 nonskid mat ▪ 1 wedge

Optional Props: 1 wall ▪ 2 blocks

Downward-Facing Dog Pose is practiced here with a wedge under the heels (Figure 12). Place a wedge at the far end of a nonskid mat so that the thin edge faces the front end of the mat. (To prevent the wedge from sliding, place your mat and wedge at the base of a wall.) Come onto your hands and knees with your toes turned under and your feet directly in front of the wedge. With an inhalation, lengthen your arms and

12. DOWNWARD-FACING DOG POSE,
WITH HEELS SUPPORTED

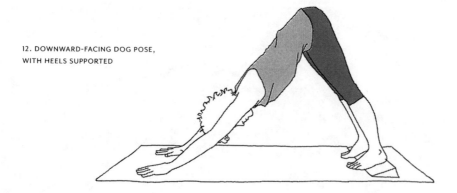

press your big toes into the mat. With an exhalation, lift your pelvis away from your rib cage and straighten your legs. Lengthen your lower calf muscles away from your Achilles tendons as you rest your heels on the wedge.

Adjust your feet, if necessary, so that your heels are fully supported by the wedge, not hanging over the back edge, and the balls of your big toes are in firm contact with the mat in front of the wedge. (If your heels do not reach the wedge because of tight shoulders or tight hamstrings, rest your heels on the wall or place two blocks on your mat to support your hands.)

Remain in the pose for about a minute. Check that your ankles are in line with the center of your hip joints and that your second metatarsals and second toes are parallel to each other. Then roll your first metatarsals toward your inner foot, and lift your inner anklebones away from the inner corner of your heels. At the same time, broaden your heels and lengthen your lower calf muscles away from the Achilles tendons. To come out of the pose, bend your knees, lower your shinbones, and rest your torso on your thighs before coming up.

Practice Notes. In Downward-Facing Dog Pose, keep your shinbones lifting away from your ankle joints by lengthening your lower calf muscles away from the Achilles tendons. When you push your shinbones down into your ankle joints, you compress the joint and weaken your arches. As a general rule: To create space in a joint, move the bones that form the joint away from each other, not toward each other. In Downward-Facing Dog, the heels broaden and move down, but the shinbones relax and lift.

Mountain Pose

TADASANA

▼ ▼ ▼ ▼ ▼ ▼ ▼ ▼ ▼ ▼ ▼

aligns the feet ▪ strengthens the metatarsals and broadens
the balls of the feet ▪ balances the inner and outer arches

Prop: 1 nonskid mat

Optional Prop: 1 wedge

Stand in Mountain Pose on a nonskid mat with your feet slightly apart, so that your ankles are vertically in line with the center of your hip joints (Figure 13). Check that your second metatarsals and second toes are parallel to each other. Then lengthen your metatarsals and broaden the balls of your feet by moving the neck of your little toes away from the ball of your big toes. Check that your weight is distributed evenly around the whole circumference of your heels so that the fleshy pad of your heels feels broad and cushiony.

Remain in Mountain Pose for half a minute. Continue to broaden the balls of your feet, as you lengthen your outer metatarsals toward your toes. Roll your first metatarsals toward the inner foot, but at the same time lift your inner anklebones away from the inner corner of your heels. Check that your inner and outer arches are evenly lifted. Allow your spine to lengthen.

Return to Mountain Pose after every standing pose to realign your feet and check your balance.

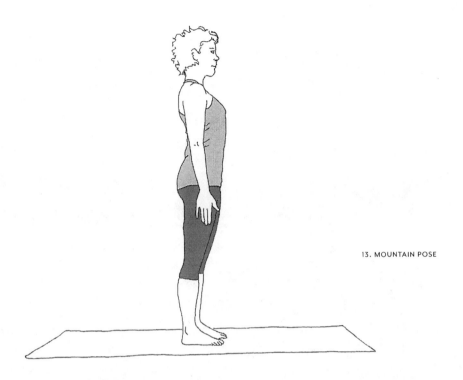

13. MOUNTAIN POSE

Practice Notes. If you have bunions or incipient bunions, remember to distribute your weight evenly around the whole circumference of the ball of the big toe, to bring your big toe and first metatarsal into better alignment.

If you have hammertoes, or otherwise need to lengthen and straighten your toes, you can practice Mountain Pose with a wedge under your toes, as pictured for Chair Pose (page 61). Place the wedge under your feet so that the balls of the feet are on the wedge and the necks of the toes are supported by the thin edge of the wedge. Use the pressure of your toes against the wedge to lengthen your toes and widen the balls of your feet.

STANDING POSE

Tree Pose

VRKSASANA

▼ ▼ ▼ ▼ ▼ ▼ ▼ ▼ ▼ ▼ ▼

improves balance ▪ strengthens the inner thighs

Props: 1 nonskid mat ▪ 1 wall

Tree Pose is practiced here by resting the knee of the bent leg on the wall (Figure 14).

Place a nonskid mat along the base of a wall. Then stand in Mountain Pose (page · 52) with your right side toward the wall, about 15 to 18 inches away from the wall. Check that your second metatarsals are parallel to the wall. With an inhalation, shift your weight onto your left foot, and gently bend your right knee as you come up onto the toes of your right foot. (If necessary, you can bring your right hand onto the wall to steady yourself.) With an exhalation, lift your right leg and take hold of your right shinbone with your left hand. Place your right foot as high as possible on your inner left thigh so that your right heel is near your left sitting bone, and let your right knee rest on the wall.

Now bring your hands to the top of your pelvis, and check that your pelvis is facing directly forward. Your right knee will not be in line with your pelvis but on the wall a few inches forward of the pelvis. Then bring your hands together in *namaste* (prayer position) in front of your breastbone, and turn the mounds of your thumbs toward your inner wrists. Broaden your palms, lengthen your fingers, and allow your shoulders to relax.

Remain in Tree Pose for about a minute. Firm the front of your left foot by moving the neck of the little toe away from the ball of the big toe. Press your right heel against your inner left thigh, and firm your inner left thigh against the heel. At the same time, lengthen your inner right thigh from your right groin toward your inner right knee.

To come out of the pose, with an inhalation, place your right hand on the wall, and with an exhalation, release your right leg and return to Mountain Pose. Repeat to the other side.

Practice Notes. The way we use our hands in prayer position can give us insight into how to best work with the feet. If you stand in Mountain Pose and push your hands against each other in namaste, the ridge of your shoulders will tighten and hunch up toward your ears. On the other hand, if you broaden your palms and lengthen your fingers against each other, your shoulders will relax and your upper arms descend.

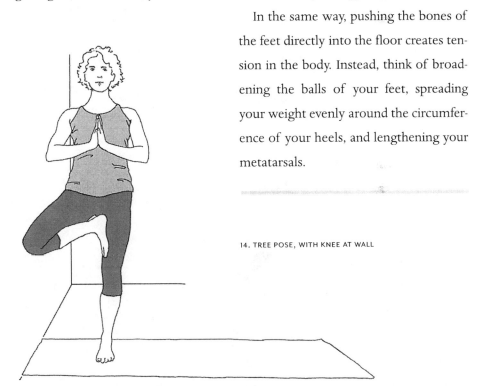

In the same way, pushing the bones of the feet directly into the floor creates tension in the body. Instead, think of broadening the balls of your feet, spreading your weight evenly around the circumference of your heels, and lengthening your metatarsals.

14. TREE POSE, WITH KNEE AT WALL

STANDING POSE

Toe-Holding Pose

PADANGUSTHASANA

▼ ▼ ▼ ▼ ▼ ▼ ▼ ▼ ▼ ▼ ▼

aligns and strengthens the big toes ▪ beneficial for those
with bunions or incipient bunions

Props: 1 nonskid mat ▪ 1 strap

Toe-Holding Pose is practiced here with a strap around the big toes (Figures 15 and 15A).

Stand in Mountain Pose (page 52) with your feet hip-width apart and your second metatarsals parallel to each other. Check that the balls of your big toes turn slightly in and that your weight is distributed evenly around the whole circumference

15. TOE-HOLDING POSE,
WITH STRAP AROUND BIG TOES

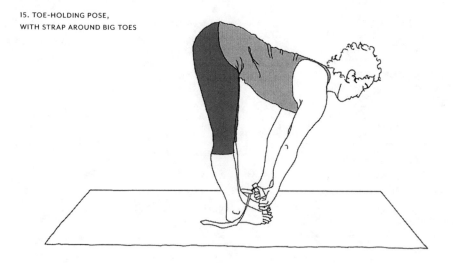

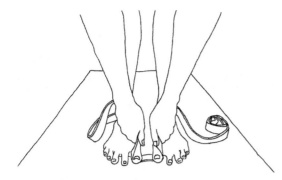

15A. STRAP AROUND BIG TOES: DETAIL

of your heels. With an inhalation, roll your first metatarsals toward the inner foot, and lengthen your outer metatarsals toward the toes. With an exhalation, keep your inner and outer arches evenly lifted as you come forward. Now take the strap with both hands and loop it around your big toes. Hold the strap between your index fingers and your thumbs. As you lift the strap away from the floor, press your index fingers into the strap to bring your big toes in line with your first metatarsals.

Remain in Toe-Holding Pose with a strap around your big toes for about a minute. Keep your arms extended, your spine long, and your head lifted. Press the strap against your big toes to bring them parallel to each other. To avoid hyperextending your knees, keep the skin of the heels moving back. Then firm the inner corner of the balls of the big toes, and lengthen the neck of the big toes forward from there. At the same time, firm the inner corners of your heels, and lift your lower calf muscles away from your Achilles tendons.

To come out of the pose, first release hold of the strap. With an inhalation, raise your torso, and with an exhalation, return to Mountain Pose.

Practice Notes. If you practice Toe-Holding Pose without a strap, wrap your index fingers around the neck of your big toes. Do not use your index fingers to pull your big toes away from the floor. Instead, press the neck of your big toes firmly against your index fingers, and lengthen your big toes away from your first metatarsals.

Extended Triangle Pose

UTTHITA TRIKONASANA

▼ ▼ ▼ ▼ ▼ ▼ ▼ ▼ ▼ ▼ ▼

the support of the wall stabilizes the back leg and improves balance

▪ recommended when recovering from a sprained ankle or foot injury

Caution: If you feel pain in your inner knees when practicing this pose, follow the special instructions in the Practice Notes.

Props: 1 nonskid mat ▪ 1 wall

Optional Prop: 1 block

Extended Triangle Pose is practiced here with the heel of the back foot supported by a wall (Figure 16).

Spread a nonskid mat with one end at the base of a wall. Then stand with your feet 4 to 4½ feet apart and your left foot against the wall. Turn your left foot in so that the balls of your left foot are parallel to the long edge of the mat and your outer left heel is touching the wall. Turn your right foot out so that the second metatarsal is parallel to the long edge of the mat and the ball of the big toe is turned slightly in.

With an inhalation, place your left hand on your outer left hip and raise your right arm to shoulder level. With an exhalation, press your outer left heel against the wall, and lengthen the outer metatarsals of your right foot toward your toes, as you extend your torso over your right leg. Bring your right hand to the floor, and raise your left arm toward the ceiling. (If your right hand doesn't reach the floor easily, place a block by your outer right ankle for support.)

In Extended Triangle Pose, notice whether your weight falls onto the outer edge or inner edge of your front foot (the right foot). To balance the inner and outer foot, lengthen your outer metatarsals toward the toes, broaden the balls of the foot, and lift your inner anklebone away from the inner corner of your heel. Check that your inner and outer arches are evenly lifted.

To adjust the back foot (the left foot), press your outer heel into the wall, and lift your inner anklebone away from the inner corner of your heel. Relax the bones at the top of your foot, and release the front of your ankle joint. Roll your outer metatarsals toward the outer foot and your first metatarsal toward the inner foot so that the inner and outer arches lift evenly.

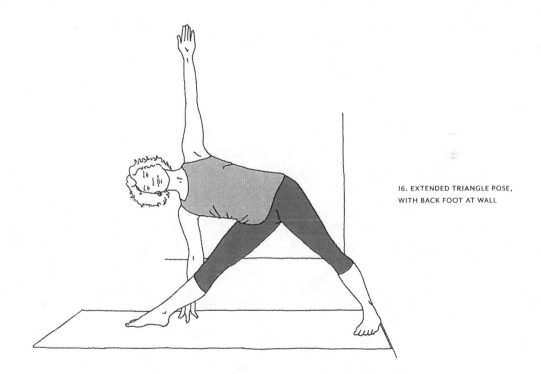

16. EXTENDED TRIANGLE POSE, WITH BACK FOOT AT WALL

Remain in Extended Triangle Pose for another half minute. To come out of the pose, lengthen the outer metatarsals of your right foot toward the toes, and press the outer left heel into the wall with an inhalation, as you lift your torso to an upright position. With an exhalation, lower your arms and repeat to the other side.

Practice Notes. You can use the wall to support your back leg in other asymmetrical standing poses, such as Warrior Pose II (page 63), Extended Side-Angle Pose (page 68), and Warrior Pose I (page 77).

If you feel pain in your inner right knee when practicing Extended Triangle Pose to the right, come out of the pose and begin again. If your right knee turns in when your right foot points forward, you may need to change the placement of your foot. Instead of aligning the second metatarsal with the long edge of the mat, turn your right foot out until the center of your knee points forward, to avoid compression of the inner knee.

STANDING POSE
Chair Pose
UTKATASANA

▼ ▼ ▼ ▼ ▼ ▼ ▼ ▼ ▼ ▼ ▼

lengthens and strengthens the toes ▪ increases flexibility of the ankle joints ▪ lengthens the Achilles tendons ▪ counters hyperextension of the knees ▪ relieves plantar fasciitis ▪ recommended for those with curled or hammer toes but beneficial for all

Props: 1 nonskid mat ▪ 1 wedge

Chair Pose is practiced here with a wedge under the toes (Figures 17 and 17A).

Place a wedge near the front of your mat with the thin edge pointing back. Stand in Mountain Pose (page 52) with your feet hip-width apart and your toes supported

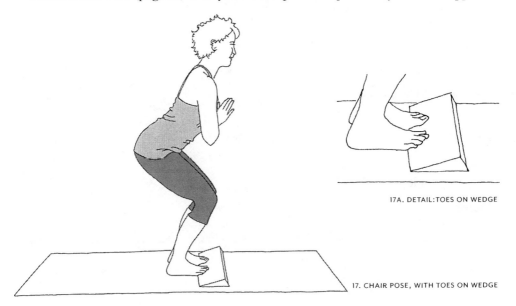

17A. DETAIL: TOES ON WEDGE

17. CHAIR POSE, WITH TOES ON WEDGE

by the thin edge of the wedge, so that the tips of your toes are higher than the necks of your toes. Check that your second metatarsals are parallel to each other and that the balls of your big toes are close to but not on the wedge. With an inhalation, bring your hands together in *namaste* (prayer position) in front of your breastbone, and press the necks of your toes against the wedge. With an exhalation, release the top of your shinbones forward as you bend your knees. Release your kneecaps away from your knee joints, and soften the muscles at the back of your knees.

Remain in Chair Pose for half a minute. Relax the tarsal bones at the top of your feet to release the front of your ankle joints. Let your lower calf muscles release away from your heels to lengthen the Achilles tendons. Shift your weight onto the front of your feet, but let the skin of your heels move back. Ideally, you will feel a deeper stretch of the Achilles tendons, more flexibility in your ankle joints, and a deeper bend of your knees.

To come out of the pose, press the necks of your toes against the wedge, lift your thighbones away from your shinbones to straighten your legs, and return to Mountain Pose.

Practice Notes. You can use a wedge under your toes in other symmetrical standing poses, such as Mountain Pose and Standing Forward Bend (page 66), to strengthen and lengthen your toes.

STANDING POSE
Warrior Pose II
VIRABHADRASANA II

▼ ▼ ▼ ▼ ▼ ▼ ▼ ▼ ▼ ▼ ▼ ▼

lengthens and strengthens the toes ▪ recommended
for those with curled or hammer toes

Props: 1 nonskid mat ▪ 1 wedge

Warrior Pose II is practiced here with a wedge under the toes of the bent leg (Figures 18 and 18A).

Stand in Mountain Pose (page 52) on your nonskid mat with your feet 4 to 4½ feet apart. Turn your left foot in so that the balls of the foot are parallel to the long edge

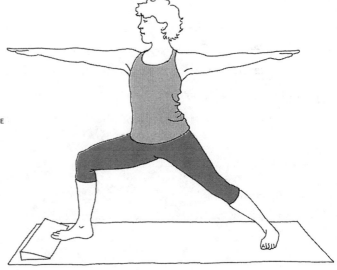

18. WARRIOR POSE II, WITH TOES ON WEDGE

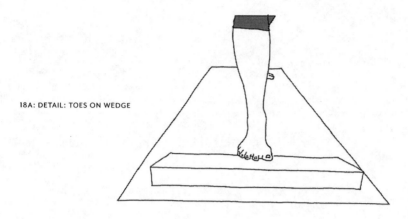

18A: DETAIL: TOES ON WEDGE

of the mat. Turn your right foot out so that the second metatarsal is parallel to the long edge of the mat. Place the thin edge of a wedge under the toes of your right foot so that the balls of the foot remain on the mat but all five toes are supported by the wedge. (To accomplish this, you may need to turn the wedge at an angle to the frontal plane of the foot.)

With an inhalation, broaden your left heel and raise your arms out to the side at shoulder level. With an exhalation, lengthen the toes of your right foot against the wedge as you bend your right knee.

Remain in Warrior Pose II with your toes on a wedge for about a minute. With your left or extended leg, broaden the balls of your left foot, and lift your lower calf muscle away from the circumference of your heel. With your right or bent leg, broaden the circumference of the ball of your big toe as you lengthen the other toes against the wedge.

To come out of the pose, with an inhalation, press the necks of the toes of your right foot evenly against the wedge as you straighten your right leg. With an exhalation, lower your arms, and then repeat to the other side.

Practice Notes. You can use a wedge under the toes in other asymmetrical standing poses, such as Tree Pose (page 54), Extended Triangle Pose (page 58), Extended Side-Angle Pose (page 68), Half Moon Pose (page 74), and Warrior I Pose (page 77) to facilitate the lengthening and strengthening of the toes.

STANDING POSES

Standing Forward Bend

UTTANASANA

▼ ▼ ▼ ▼ ▼ ▼ ▼ ▼ ▼ ▼ ▼ ▼

enhances the lateral range of motion of the ankle joints
▪ improves balance by strengthening the feet ▪ recommended for those
with weak arches or unstable ankles ▪ excellent preparation for
balancing poses such as Tree Pose and Half Moon Pose

Props: 1 nonskid mat ▪ 2 wedges

Optional Props: 2 blocks

Standing Forward Bend is practiced here with your feet on wedges (Figures 19 and 19A).

Place two wedges lengthwise on a nonskid mat, with the high edges touching. Then stand on the wedges in Mountain Pose, with feet hip-width apart and your sec-

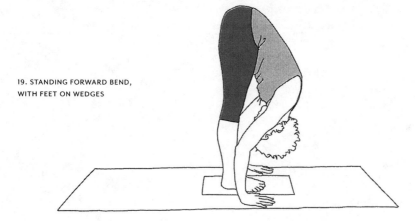

19. STANDING FORWARD BEND,
WITH FEET ON WEDGES

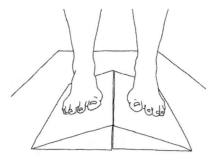

19A. DETAIL: FEET ON WEDGES

ond metatarsals parallel to each other. Check that the balls of your big toes are turned slightly in. With an inhalation, place your hands on your hips and lengthen the outer edges of your feet. With an exhalation, lift your lower calf muscles away from your heels as you extend your torso forward. Place your hands on the floor by the sides of the feet, and release your head and neck. (If your hands do not reach the floor easily, use a block to support each hand.)

Remain in Standing Forward Bend with your feet on wedges for about a minute. Widen the balls of your feet by moving the little toe away from the ball of the big toe. Check that your weight is evenly distributed around the circumference of the heels, and let the soles of your feet conform to the surface of the wedges.

To come out of the pose, bring your hands onto your hips. With an inhalation, lengthen the outer edges of your feet against the wedges as you lift your torso to an upright position. With an exhalation, step off the wedges onto your mat and stand quietly in Mountain Pose. Observe the strength and balance of your feet and legs.

Practice Notes. When your weight is not distributed evenly around the whole circumference of your heel, lift the heel slightly away from the wedge, find the very center of the heel, and then bring the heel down again. When you rest on the very center of the heel, your weight will be more evenly balanced around the circumference.

Extended Side-Angle Pose

UTTHITA PARSVAKONASANA

▼ ▼ ▼ ▼ ▼ ▼ ▼ ▼ ▼ ▼ ▼

strengthens the inner foot ▪ relaxes the groins
▪ aligns the pelvis and legs ▪ recommended for those who stand
on the outer edges of their feet and those with tight
or injured groin muscles

Props: 1 nonskid mat ▪ 1 wedge

Optional Prop: 1 block

Extended Side-Angle Pose is practiced here with the inner foot of the bent leg on a wedge (Figures 20 and 20A).

Stand in Mountain Pose (page 52) on your nonskid mat, and bring your feet 4 to 4½ feet apart. Turn your right foot out so that the second metatarsal is parallel to the long edge of the mat. Then place a wedge lengthwise under your inner right foot so that your second metatarsal and inner half of the heel are supported by the thin edge of the wedge. Then turn your left foot in so that the balls of the foot are parallel to the long edge of the mat.

With an inhalation, lift your lower left calf muscle away from your heel, and raise your arms out to the side at shoulder level. With an exhalation, lengthen the outer metatarsals of your right foot, as you bend your right knee and extend your torso over your right thigh. Place your right hand on the floor by your outer right ankle, and swing your left arm overhead in line with your outer left rib cage. (Use a block to support your right hand if you cannot reach the floor easily.)

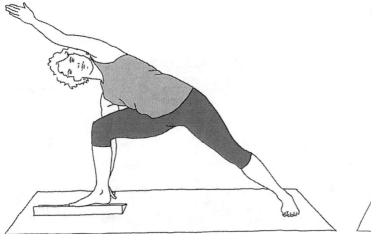 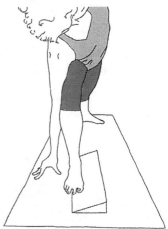

20. EXTENDED SIDE-ANGLE POSE, WITH INNER FOOT ON WEDGE   20 A. DETAIL: INNER FOOT ON WEDGE

Remain in Extended Side-Angle Pose with your inner foot on a wedge for about a minute. Take some time to observe your right leg and foot. Is your right thighbone in line with the frontal plane of your body? Does the head of your right thighbone feel centered in your right hip socket, or does it feel jammed? Does your right groin area feel tight and compressed or relaxed and broad?

When you are ready, come out of the pose with an inhalation, broadening the balls of your right foot as you straighten your right leg and raise your torso. With an exhalation, lower your arms and repeat the pose to the other side.

Practice Notes. If you have never practiced Extended Side-Angle Pose with your inner foot on a wedge, try doing the pose without a wedge immediately before. In this way, you can tell what difference the prop makes for you and whether it is beneficial. Do not continue using a prop if you feel it has a negative effect.

STANDING POSE

Wide-Leg Standing Forward Bend

PRASARITA PADOTTANASANA

▼ ▼ ▼ ▼ ▼ ▼ ▼ ▼ ▼ ▼ ▼

balances the inner and outer ankle joints ▪ relieves strain on the
outer ankle and outer calf ▪ creates space in the hip joints ▪ recommended
if you have sprained your ankle or feel a burning
sensation in your outer calf

Props: 1 nonskid mat ▪ 2 wedges

Optional Props: 2 blocks

Wide-Leg Standing Forward Bend is practiced here with the feet on wedges (Figure 21).

Place two wedges on your mat, 4 to 4½ feet apart. Align the wedges parallel to each other, with the thin edges facing in. Fold the ends of your mat over the wedges to

21. WIDE-LEG STANDING FORWARD
BEND, WITH FEET ON WEDGES
(FOLD ENDS OF MAT OVER WEDGES)

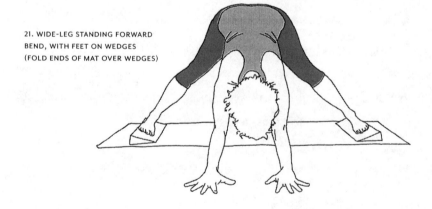

prevent them from sliding. (If your mat is not long enough, place the wedges closer together.) Then stand on your mat with your feet just inside the wedges.

With an inhalation, roll your outer metatarsals toward your outer feet and your first metatarsals toward your inner feet. With an exhalation, extend your torso forward, and place your hands on the floor directly beneath your shoulders. Use your arms for support as you step first one foot and then the other onto the wedges. Position your feet so that your second metatarsals are parallel to each other and the balls of your big toes turn slightly in. When your feet and legs feel steady, extend your arms forward, and lengthen the sides of your chest, as for Downward-Facing Dog Pose. (If your shoulders or hamstrings are tight, place your hands on blocks, and lift the sides of your chest away from your elbows.)

Remain in Wide-Leg Standing Forward Bend with your feet on wedges for another minute. Roll your outer metatarsals toward your outer foot, and broaden the circumference of the balls of your big toes. At the same time, lift your inner anklebones away from the inner corners of your heels, and lengthen the sides of your chest.

To come out of the pose, walk your hands back until they are directly beneath your shoulders. Keep your arms extended and your spine long as you step off the wedges, and then walk or spring your feet together. With an inhalation, place your hands onto your hips, and lengthen your spine. With an exhalation, lift your torso and return to Mountain Pose.

Practice Notes. If you feel a burning sensation on your outer calves when you practice Wide-Leg Standing Forward Bend without wedges, you are probably sickling your feet and stressing your outer ankle joints. When you use wedges under the feet, your ankle joints are restored to a more neutral position, which not only relieves any discomfort in your outer calves but also brings freedom of movement to the hip joints, so that you feel a deeper and healthier stretch of the hamstrings.

STANDING POSE

Standing Forward Bend

UTTANASANA

▼ ▼ ▼ ▼ ▼ ▼ ▼ ▼ ▼ ▼ ▼

activates the arches ▪ strengthens the inner corner
of the heels ▪ balances the inner and outer foot ▪ recommended
for those with weak arches but beneficial for everyone

Props: 1 nonskid mat ▪ 1 strap

Standing Forward Bend is practiced here with a strap around the arches (Figures 22 and 22A).

Make a large loop with your strap, about 3 feet in diameter. Stand on your mat in Mountain Pose with your feet hip-width apart (page 52). With an inhalation, firm the inner corners of your heels, and lift your inner and outer arches evenly. With an exha-

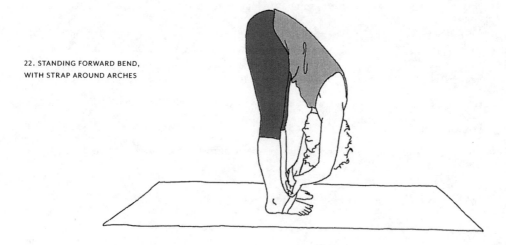

22. STANDING FORWARD BEND,
WITH STRAP AROUND ARCHES

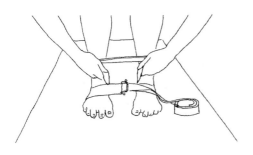

22A. DETAIL: STRAP AROUND ARCHES

lation, broaden the balls of your feet and lift your lower calf muscles away from your Achilles tendons as you lengthen your torso forward. Then loop your strap around your arches with the buckle uppermost. Hold the buckle of the strap upright with your left hand. With your right hand, reach down between the arches from behind the buckle, and draw the lower part of the strap away from the floor. Let go of the buckle so that the upper part of the strap is firm across the top of the feet and the lower part of the strap supports the arches and presses against the inner corner of the heels.

Remain in Standing Forward Bend with a strap around your arches for about a minute. Check that your second metatarsals are parallel to each other and that the balls of your big toes turn slightly in. Bend your elbows out to the side, and with your hands draw the strap firmly against the inner corners of your heels, and simultaneously roll your first metatarsals toward your inner foot. Lengthen your outer metatarsals toward your toes, and lift your lower calf muscles away from the Achilles tendons. Let your spine release into the forward bend.

To come out of the pose, remove the strap from around your feet. With an inhalation, bring your hands onto your hips, and lift your torso to an upright position. With an exhalation, release your arms and return to Mountain Pose.

Practice Notes. When you practice Standing Forward Bend without a strap under your arches, use the tips of your index fingers to press against the inner corner of your heels. Then firm the inner corner of your heels, and lift your lower calf muscles away from your Achilles tendons.

STANDING POSE

Half Moon Pose

ARHDA CHANDRASANA

strengthens the front of the foot ▪ balances inner and outer arches
▪ avoids hyperextension of the knee

Props: 1 nonskid mat ▪ 1 block

Optional Prop: 1 wall

Half Moon Pose is practiced here with your hand on a block directly beneath your shoulder (Figure 23).

Stand in Mountain Pose (page 52) on a nonskid mat, and step your feet 4 to 4½ feet apart. Turn your left foot in so that the balls of your left foot are parallel to the long edge of the mat. Turn your right foot out so that your second metatarsal is parallel to the long edge of the mat and the ball of your big toe turns slightly in. Place a block on the mat by your outer right foot.

With an inhalation, raise your arms to shoulder level. With an exhalation, bend your right knee by releasing your shinbone forward. With another inhalation, lift your left heel off the floor, and shift your weight onto the front of your right foot. With an exhalation, lift your right thighbone to straighten your right leg, and bring your right hand onto the block directly beneath your shoulder. Your spine should be parallel to the floor. (If you are unable to maintain your balance, stand with your back resting against a wall for support.)

Remain in Half Moon Pose for about a minute. On your standing leg, lengthen the outer metatarsals of your right foot toward the toes, and lift your outer right arch.

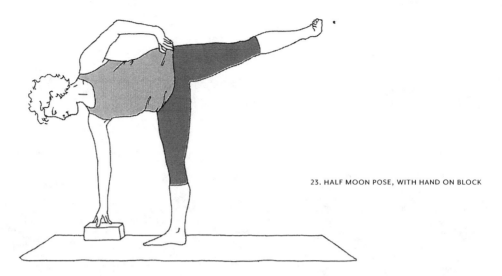

23. HALF MOON POSE, WITH HAND ON BLOCK

At the same time, lift your inner right anklebone away from the inner corner of your right heel. Spread your weight evenly around the whole circumference of the ball of your big toe. With your raised leg, broaden the balls of your left foot, and firm the inner corner of your left heel.

To come out of the pose, bend your right knee by pressing the top of your right shinbone forward. At the same time, relax the front of the ankle joint, and lengthen your Achilles tendon away from your right heel. Keep your left foot active as you lower your left leg, and broaden the front of your left foot as soon as it touches the floor. Then, with an inhalation, lift your right thighbone to straighten your right leg, and bring your torso to an upright position. With an exhalation, lower your arms, and repeat to the other side.

Practice Notes. As a general rule in standing poses, bend your knee from the shinbone, but straighten your leg from the thighbone. Following this simple rule helps to avoid hyperextending your knee, especially in Half Moon Pose.

To bend your knee, release the grip of your kneecap and soften the muscles at the back of your knee as you press the top of the shinbone forward. The thighbone slightly resists the movement of the shinbone. Relax the front of the ankle joint, and lengthen the Achilles tendon to bring more weight onto the front of the foot and deepen the bend of the knee.

To straighten the leg, move the skin of the heel back as you lift the head of the thighbone into the center of your hip joint. Let the shinbone resist the movement of the thighbone. When the leg is almost straight, firm the inner knee and spread your weight evenly around the circumference of the ball of the big toe.

STANDING POSE
Warrior Pose I
VIRABHADRASANA I

▼ ▼ ▼ ▼ ▼ ▼ ▼ ▼ ▼ ▼ ▼ ▼

provides support for the heel of the extended leg ▪ relieves compression
of the ankle joint and strengthens the inner knees ▪ recommended if
the heel of your extended leg comes off the floor in this pose
or if your inner arch collapses

Props: 1 nonskid mat ▪ 1 wall ▪ 1 wedge

Warrior Pose I is practiced here with a wedge supporting the heel of the extended leg (Figures 24 and 24A).

Spread a nonskid mat with one end at the base of
a wall. Place a wedge on the mat with the high edge
against the wall. Then stand on the mat in Mountain
Pose (page 52) with your back
to the wall. Bring your right
leg forward so that the second
metatarsal of your right foot is
parallel to the long edge of the
mat. Bring your left leg back,
and turn your left foot out

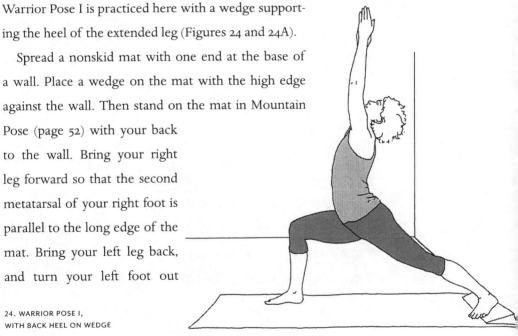

24. WARRIOR POSE I,
WITH BACK HEEL ON WEDGE

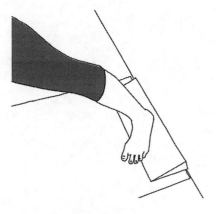

24A. DETAIL: BACK HEEL ON WEDGE

about 30 degrees. Place your left foot on the wedge so that both your heel and the ball of the little toe are supported by the wedge but the ball of your big toe remains on the mat. With an inhalation, raise your arms overhead. With an exhalation, bend your right knee and press your right shinbone forward, softening the muscles at the back of the knee.

Remain in Warrior Pose I for about a minute. With your left foot, broaden the neck of your little toe away from the ball of your big toe. Spread your weight evenly around the circumference of your left heel, and lift your lower calf muscle away from the Achilles tendon. With your right foot, lengthen the outer metatarsals toward the toes, and broaden the balls of your foot.

To come out of the pose, with an inhalation, lengthen the outer metatarsals of your right foot toward the toes as you lift your right thighbone and straighten your right leg. With an exhalation, lower your arms, return to Mountain Pose, and repeat to the other side.

Practice Notes. When practicing Warrior Pose I without a wedge under your back heel, it is more difficult to keep the lower shinbone lifting away from the ankle joint of the extended leg. When practicing the pose to the right, lift the outer arch of your right foot, firm down from the inner corner of the right heel, and lift up from the inner right anklebone. With your extended left leg, roll the outer metatarsals toward the outer left foot, firm down from the inner corner of your left heel, and lift up from your inner left anklebone. Lifting your inner anklebones away from the inner corners of your heels keeps the inner arches from collapsing.

BACK BEND

Camel Pose

USTRASANA

▼ ▼ ▼ ▼ ▼ ▼ ▼ ▼ ▼ ▼ ▼ ▼

takes pressure off the ankle joints ▪ releases the hip joints
▪ for those with high arches, prevents the feet from cramping

Caution: Do not practice this pose if you experience knee pain. If you have a neck injury or feel discomfort in your neck, keep your head lifted throughout this pose.

Props: 1 nonskid mat ▪ 1 blanket ▪ 1 wedge ▪ 1 block

Optional Prop: 1 bolster

Camel Pose is practiced here with the top of the feet on a wedge (Figure 25).

Spread a folded blanket on your mat to support your knees and shins. Lay a wedge near the far end of the blanket, with the high edge facing forward. Place a block flat and lengthwise on the wedge, with one end of the block in line with the high edge of the wedge. Kneel on the blanket, with the top of your feet on the wedge and your inner feet pressing against the block. With an inhalation, bring

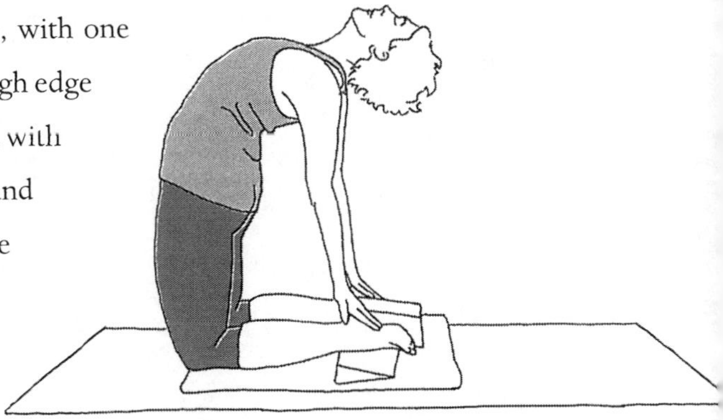

25. CAMEL POSE, WITH FEET ON WEDGE

your hands onto your hips, and lift your rib cage away from your pelvis. With an exhalation, extend your arms and take hold of your heels. (If you have difficulty reaching your heels, place a bolster across your ankles to support your hands.)

Remain in Camel Pose with your feet on a wedge for about a minute. Relax the bones at the top of your feet, and lengthen your metatarsals so that your toes lift away from the floor. Feel how the action of your feet creates length at the front of your thighs and space in your hip joints. Lift your rib cage away from your pelvis, and let your head drop back only if you feel no strain in your neck.

To come out of the pose, lengthen your front thighs and lift your rib cage with an inhalation. With an exhalation, sit back on your heels, raise your head, and rest with your hands on your thighs. Repeat the pose two or three times.

Practice Notes. When you practice Camel Pose without a wedge under the feet, still use a block between your feet so that your ankles, knees, and hip joints are all aligned. Lengthen your first metatarsals against the block, and firm the inner corners of the balls of your big toes.

TWISTING POSE

Simple Seated Twist II

BHARADVAJASANA II

▼ ▼ ▼ ▼ ▼ ▼ ▼ ▼ ▼ ▼ ▼ ▼

balances the inner and outer foot ▪ reduces strain on
the knee joint ▪ creates space in the hip joints

Caution: Do not practice this pose if you
experience knee pain.

Props: 1 nonskid mat ▪ 1 blanket
▪ 1 facecloth

Optional Prop: 1 strap

Simple Seated Twist II is practiced here with a
folded facecloth supporting the inner foot of
the leg in Hero position (Figures 26 and 26A).

Sit on a blanket in Staff Pose (page 86) with
your legs extended. Fold a facecloth over twice
to form a long, narrow strip about 3 inches wide
and 12 inches long. Place the facecloth lengthwise by your outer right hip. Bend your right
knee, and place the top of your right foot along-

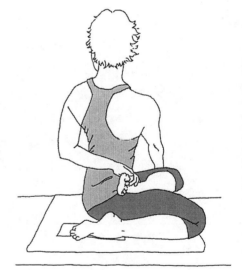

26. SIMPLE SEATED TWIST II, WITH INNER FOOT SUPPORTED

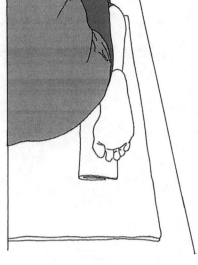

26A. DETAIL: INNER FOOT SUPPORTED

side your outer right hip, as for Hero Pose (page 84), so that the facecloth supports the inner foot and the outer foot drops to the blanket. Then bend your left knee, and rest the top of your left foot on your right thigh, as for Lotus Pose. (If the Lotus position is difficult for you, place the top of your left foot on the blanket by your inner right thigh, as for Head-of-the-Knee Pose (page 88).

Bring your left arm behind your back, and take hold of your left foot. (If you are unable to take hold of the foot, use a strap around the foot or ankle.) Place your right hand on your outer left leg, with your arm extended. Relax your lower abdomen, and lift and turn your upper abdomen to the left.

Remain in Simple Seated Twist II with your inner right foot supported for about a minute. Lengthen the outer metatarsals of your left foot, and lift your left inner ankle-bone away from the inner corner of your heel. Keep your diaphragm soft and broad as you lift and turn your upper abdomen away from your lower abdomen. To come out of the pose, release your arms and legs, and repeat the pose to the other side.

Practice Notes. If you practice Simple Seated Twist II without a prop under your foot, take a few moments to observe the balance of the pose. How does the top of your foot make contact with the blanket? Do you feel the pressure more on your inner foot or on your outer foot? Is your sitting bone on that side lifting or descending? What is the feeling in your knee and hip joint?

Compare this with how you feel when you practice Simple Seated Twist II with your inner right foot supported. The weight on the top of your right foot should now be more evenly distributed between your inner and outer foot. This in turn brings your right shinbone and thighbone into better alignment, reducing any strain on your right knee and allowing your right hip joint to relax, so that your right sitting bone comes closer to the floor.

Hero Pose

VIRASANA

▼ ▼ ▼ ▼ ▼ ▼ ▼ ▼ ▼ ▼ ▼ ▼

relieves discomfort in the ankles and feet ▪ prevents feet from
cramping ▪ may relieve knee pain ▪ recommended for
those with high arches or stiff ankles

Caution: Do not practice this pose if you continue to experience knee pain.

Props: 1 nonskid mat ▪ 1 blanket ▪ 2 facecloths

Optional Prop: 1 block

Hero Pose is practiced here with support under the ankles (Figure 27).

Place a folded blanket on your nonskid mat to support your shins and feet. Kneel on the blanket with your thighs parallel and your feet hip-width apart, and sit back between your heels. (If your pelvis doesn't reach the floor easily, use a block under your sitting bones.)

Make two firm rolls with your facecloths by folding each facecloth in half and rolling it tightly from the narrow end. With an inhalation, lean forward with your torso, and lift your ankles away from the floor. With an exhalation, slide the rolled facecloths between your ankles and the blanket, and lift your torso to an upright position. (If you experience discomfort or cramping in your feet, increase the height of the roll under your ankles. Make sure that the rolls are supporting the front of your ankle joints, not your lower shinbones.)

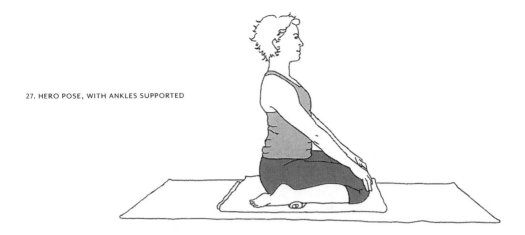

27. HERO POSE, WITH ANKLES SUPPORTED

Place your palms on your thighs just above your knees, with your arms extended. Press the heels of your hands toward your knees, to encourage the front of your thighs to lengthen. At the same time, relax the bones at the top of your feet, and lengthen your outer metatarsals toward the toes. Remain in this position for a minute or two.

To come out of the pose, lean forward onto your hands, lift your ankles away from the floor, and remove the rolled facecloths. Then cross your ankles and sit back on your sitting bones. Place your hands by the sides of your pelvis, extend your legs, and sit in Staff Pose (page 86) for half a minute to restore the circulation in your legs.

Practice Notes. A teacher can tell when a student needs a support under the ankles in Hero Pose by looking at the color of the skin at the back of the ankle. If the skin is blanched and yellowish, the ankle joint is jammed and overworked. In this case, placing a support under the ankle restores circulation, and the skin at the back of the ankle resumes its natural color.

Staff Pose

DANDASANA

▼ ▼ ▼ ▼ ▼ ▼ ▼ ▼ ▼ ▼ ▼

strengthens the arches and aligns the feet and legs

Caution: Do not practice this pose if you experience knee pain.

Props: 1 nonskid mat ▪ 1 blanket ▪ 1 strap

Optional Prop: 1 wall

Staff Pose is practiced here with a strap around the arches of the feet (Figure 28).

Sit on a nonskid mat with your legs extended and your sitting bones near the edge of a folded blanket. Make a large loop with your strap, about 3 feet in diameter, and place the loop around your arches with the buckle nearest to your torso. Hold the strap in

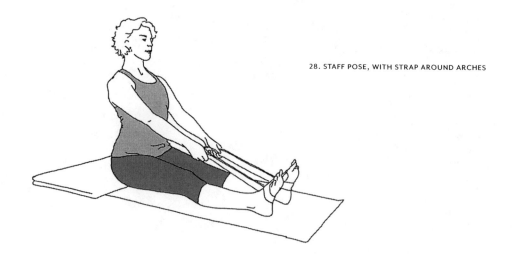

28. STAFF POSE, WITH STRAP AROUND ARCHES

place with your left hand on the buckle as you reach under the strap with your right hand and draw the strap away from your inner arches, as we do in Standing Forward Bend (page 72) with a strap around the arches.

When your strap is in place, sit in Staff Pose with your legs extended and your torso erect. Lift the inner corners of your heels away from the strap, and press your first metatarsals into the strap. (You can practice this pose with the soles of your feet against a wall to help activate your outer metatarsals and outer toes as well.)

Maintain the pose for about a minute, and then release the strap from around your feet.

Practice Notes. Return to Staff Pose with a strap around the arches after every sitting pose, to strengthen the arches and realign your feet and legs.

FORWARD BEND

Head-of-the-Knee Pose

JANU SIRSASANA

▼ ▼ ▼ ▼ ▼ ▼ ▼ ▼ ▼ ▼ ▼

recommended as a preparation for Lotus-type poses

▪ releases pressure on the outer foot and ankle of the bent leg

▪ softens the groin of the bent leg and releases the knee

Caution: Do not practice this pose if you experience knee pain.

Props: 1 nonskid mat ▪ 1 blanket ▪ 1 facecloth

Optional Props: 1 block ▪ 1 blanket ▪ 1 strap

Head-of-the-Knee Pose is practiced here with a support under the ankle of the bent leg (Figure 29).

Sit on a nonskid mat with your legs extended and your sitting bones near the edge of a folded blanket. Bend your right knee out to the side, and draw your right foot toward your right groin. (If your right knee doesn't reach the floor, support your right

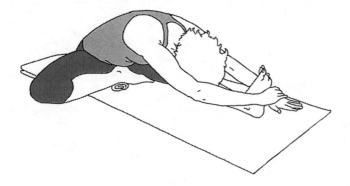

29. HEAD-OF-THE-KNEE POSE, WITH ANKLE SUPPORTED

leg with a block or a folded blanket. If your right hip joint is injured or unduly tight, support both sitting bones and the entire length of your left leg with a blanket folded in a long, narrow strip.)

For many of us, the right ankle is slightly sickled in this position, and the outer foot presses uncomfortably into the floor. To restore the ankle joint to a more neutral position and relieve any discomfort, use a prop under your right ankle. Fold a facecloth in half, and then roll it firmly from the narrow end until it is about 1½ inches in diameter. Place the roll in the hollow between your outer anklebone and your outer foot.

Ideally the roll will create space in your ankle joint, soften your right groin, and allow your right knee to descend toward the floor. (If the support feels uncomfortable, you may need to adjust the size or placement of the roll. If the roll still does not feel helpful, remove it and practice without ankle support.)

Now place your hands on the floor by the sides of your pelvis, and lengthen your spine. With an inhalation, raise your arms overhead, and firm the inner corner of your left heel. With an exhalation, draw your left groin back into your body as you lengthen your torso forward over your left leg and take hold of the left foot. (If you have difficulty reaching the foot, use a strap around the arch of the foot.)

Now adjust your extended leg: Firm the inner corner of your left heel, and turn the first metatarsal toward the inner left foot. With your bent leg, firm the inner corner of your right heel, lengthen your outer metatarsals, and broaden from your inner right groin to your outer right knee.

Remain in the pose for another minute, relaxing the bones at the top of the feet but keeping your arches active. To come out of the pose, with an inhalation, extend your arms overhead and raise your torso to a vertical position. With an exhalation, lower the arms and straighten your right leg. Repeat the pose to the other side.

Practice Notes. When you practice Head-of-the-Knee Pose without a support for your ankle, take some time to adjust the foot of your bent leg manually. When your right knee is bent, place your right hand under your right shinbone just above the ankle, and then lift and turn the shinbone away from your inner right thigh. At the same time, place your left hand around the right foot so that your fingers support the top of the foot and your thumb wraps around the arch of the foot. With your fingers, draw the bones at the top of the foot away from the ankle joint, and relax the top of your foot. With your left thumb, press firmly against the ball of your big toe to widen your metatarsals. Then place the top of your right foot on the floor by your inner left thigh, and come into Head-of-the-Knee Pose as described above.

SITTING POSE

Bound Angle Pose

BADDHA KONASANA

▼ ▼ ▼ ▼ ▼ ▼ ▼ ▼ ▼ ▼ ▼ ▼

strengthens the arches ▪ allows hip joints to relax and knees to descend

Caution: Do not practice this pose if you experience knee pain.

Props: 1 nonskid mat ▪ 1 or more blankets ▪ 1 wedge

Optional Props: 2 facecloths

Bound Angle Pose is practiced here with a wedge between the feet (Figure 30).

Sit in Staff Pose on a nonskid mat with your legs extended and your sitting bones near the edge of a folded blanket (page 86). Bend your knees out to the side, and draw

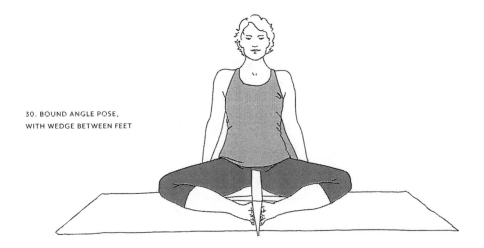

30. BOUND ANGLE POSE,
WITH WEDGE BETWEEN FEET

your feet toward your pelvis until your heels are in line with your knees. If your knees come higher than your hip joints, use at least two blankets folded in half lengthwise under your sitting bones. If your feet sickle in Bound Angle Pose, place a rolled face-cloth under each outer ankle to bring the ankle joints to a more neutral position.

Then put a wedge between the soles of your feet with the narrow edge pointing down. Place your hands on the floor behind your pelvis, and lift your rib cage away from your arms. Lean back onto your hands, widen your groins, relax your knee joints, and firm the soles of your feet against the wedge.

Maintain Bound Angle Pose with a wedge between your feet for a minute or two, keeping the rib cage lifted and the feet active. To come out of the pose, remove the wedge from between your feet, lift your knees with your hands, and straighten your legs. Sit in Staff Pose for a few breaths with your legs extended.

Practice Notes. If you have bunions or incipient bunions, use your hands to realign your big toes and first metatarsals when practicing Bound Angle Pose without a wedge between the feet. Press with your thumbs to firm the inner corners of the balls of your big toes. At the same time, use your index fingers to lift your big toes away from your second toes and bring them more in line with your first metatarsals. Broaden the balls of your big toes against each other, and lengthen the neck of your big toes.

SITTING POSE

Half Lotus Staff Pose

ARDHA PADMA DANDASANA

▼ ▼ ▼ ▼ ▼ ▼ ▼ ▼ ▼ ▼ ▼ ▼

relaxes the foot and creates space in the ankle joint
▪ takes pressure off the knee joint ▪ deeply releases the outer hip
▪ an excellent preparation for Lotus-type poses

Caution: Do not practice this pose if you experience knee pain.

Props: 1 nonskid mat ▪ 1 blanket ▪ 1 block

Optional Props: 1 blanket ▪ 1 strap

Half Lotus Staff Pose is practiced here with a support under the ankle of the bent leg (Figure 31). Sit in Staff Pose on a nonskid mat with your legs extended and your sitting bones near the edge of a folded blanket (page 86). Bend your right knee out to the side, and draw your right heel toward your inner left knee. Place a foam block lengthwise against your inner

31. HALF LOTUS STAFF POSE, WITH ANKLE SUPPORTED

left thigh. Use your right hand to lift your right shinbone and your left hand to support your right foot. Then rest your outer right anklebone on the foam block and relax the foot. Check that your right shinbone is at a right angle to your left leg.

If your right knee is higher than your right foot, you may need additional support under your right ankle. In this case, place a folded blanket between the block and your outer right shinbone so that your right foot and right knee are equidistant from the floor. This should relieve any discomfort you may feel in your right knee.

Place your hands behind your pelvis, and lengthen your arms as you lift your rib cage away from your sitting bones. Maintain this position for about a minute. With your right or bent leg, firm the inner corner of your right heel, and lengthen your outer metatarsals. With your left or extended leg, firm the inner corner of your left heel, and turn your first metatarsal toward the inner foot. (If your left leg tends to roll out, place a strap around your left foot, and press the inner corner of your left heel against the strap.)

To come out of the pose, lift your right shinbone with your right hand, remove the block with your left hand, and extend your right leg. Repeat the pose to the other side.

Practice Notes. In Half Lotus Staff Pose with the ankle supported, the foot of the bent leg is relaxed and in a neutral position, neither pronated nor supinated, which allows for more freedom of movement in the knee joint and hip joint.

SITTING POSE

Perfect Pose

SIDDHASANA

▼ ▼ ▼ ▼ ▼ ▼ ▼ ▼ ▼ ▼ ▼ ▼

recommended for long periods of sitting cross-legged
▪ relieves discomfort where the ankles and shinbones cross ▪ reduces the
likelihood of numbness in the feet and legs with prolonged sitting

Caution: Do not practice this pose if you experience knee pain.

Props: 1 nonskid mat ▪ 2 blankets ▪ 1 facecloth

Optional Props: 1 or 2 blocks

Perfect Pose is practiced here with support
between the shinbones (Figure 32).

Fold two blankets in half lengthwise,
and stack them one on top of the other on
your nonskid mat. Sit in Staff Pose (page
86) with your legs extended and your sitting bones near the edge of the blankets.
Then lean back onto your hands, bend your
knees, and rest the soles of your feet on the
floor. Lift your left shinbone with

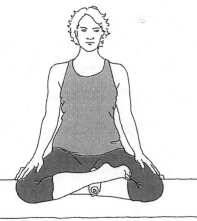

32. PERFECT POSE,
WITH SHINBONE SUPPORTED

your left hand, and use your right hand to turn the left foot out as you bring your left heel toward your right groin, and rest your outer left thigh on the floor.

Lift your right shinbone with your right hand, and use your left hand to turn the right foot out as you bring your right heel toward your left groin, and rest your right foot in the crease between your left calf and left thigh. Then fold your facecloth in half two or three times, and place it under your right shinbone just above the outer anklebone. Adjust the size and placement of the support as necessary to relieve any discomfort where the shinbones cross and to restore the right ankle joint to a neutral position.

Remain in Perfect Pose for two or three minutes. Rest your hands on your thighs, and place your elbows in line with the sides of your waist. Relax the bones at the top of your feet, and slowly lengthen your outer metatarsals. Allow your spine to gently lift. To come out of the pose, lean back on your hands, and release your legs and extend them forward, as for Staff Pose. Repeat to the other side.

Practice Notes. Perfect Pose is the perfect pose for sitting cross-legged for extended periods, such as during sitting meditation or when listening to a dharma talk. If you sit in Perfect Pose for any length of time, make sure that your knees are in contact with the floor. If not, either sit on a higher lift or support your outer thighs with blocks.

When sitting in Lotus Pose or Half Lotus Pose, it is difficult to avoid sickling, or oversupination of the feet, which weakens the ankle joint and adversely affects the knee, even with the aid of props. Perfect Pose with support between the shinbones protects the knees by balancing the inner and outer ankle joints.

INVERTED POSE

Legs-Up-the-Wall Pose
VIPARITA KARANI

▼ ▼ ▼ ▼ ▼ ▼ ▼ ▼ ▼ ▼ ▼ ▼

drains excess fluid from the feet, ankles, and legs

▪ lowers blood pressure, reduces tension, and restores energy

Caution: Do not practice this pose if you are menstruating.

Props: 1 nonskid mat ▪ 1 wall ▪ 1 bolster

Optional Prop: 1 strap

Legs-Up-the-Wall Pose is practiced here with a bolster under the pelvis (Figure 33).

Spread a nonskid mat with one end at the base of a wall. Place a bolster on the mat so it is parallel to and a few inches away from the wall. Then sit sideways on the

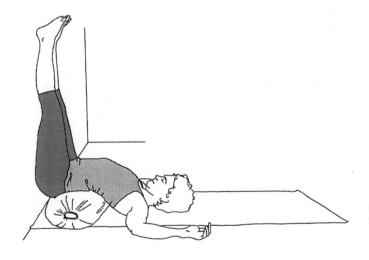

33. LEGS-UP-THE-WALL POSE,
WITH BOLSTER UNDER PELVIS

bolster with your left side against the wall. Place your hands on the floor behind you, roll your pelvis onto the bolster, and extend your legs up the wall. Lower your head and shoulders to the mat, and rest your arms out to the side.

If you feel any discomfort in your lower back, remove the bolster and rest your pelvis on the floor. If you feel any tension in your legs or groins, tie a strap around your thighs just above your knees, and relax your feet and ankles.

Remain in Legs-Up-the-Wall Pose for three to five minutes. Rest the center of your back heels against the wall so that your second metatarsals and second toes are parallel to each other. Then roll your first metatarsals in and broaden the balls of your feet. Close your eyes and soften the skin of your face. Relax your shoulders and shoulder blades. Feel the gentle movement of your rib cage with each inhalation and exhalation.

When you are ready to come out of the pose, bend your knees into your chest, and loosen the strap, if you are using one. Then slide off your bolster and roll onto your side before sitting up.

Practice Notes. When practicing Legs-Up-the-Wall with the support of a bolster, the curve of the bolster should fit the curve of your sacrum and lower lumbar spine. If your lower back does not feel supported, your bolster should be farther from the wall. In this case, bend your knees, place your feet flat on the wall, lift your pelvis, and move the bolster toward your lower back ribs. Then lower your pelvis back onto the bolster and extend your legs up the wall.

RECLINING POSE
Side-Lying Toe-Holding Pose
ANANTASANA

▼ ▼ ▼ ▼ ▼ ▼ ▼ ▼ ▼ ▼ ▼

strengthens the muscles of the arch ▪ opens the hips,
relaxes the shoulders, and lengthens the neck

Props: 1 nonskid mat ▪ 1 blanket ▪ 1 strap

Side-Lying Toe-Holding Pose is practiced here with a strap around the arch of the
raised leg (Figure 34).

Place a firmly rolled blanket lengthwise on your nonskid mat. Lie on your left side
with the blanket roll supporting the left side of your pelvis and lower back. Extend
your left arm overhead, in line with your spine. Then bend your left elbow, and place
the palm of your left hand near the base of your skull to support your head and neck.
With an inhalation, bend your right leg, and place a strap around the arch of your right

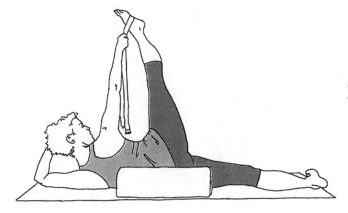

34. SIDE-LYING TOE-HOLDING POSE,
WITH STRAP AROUND ARCH

foot, close to the heel. With an exhalation, extend your right leg toward the ceiling, and lengthen your right arm.

Remain in Side-Lying Toe-Holding Pose with a strap around the arch of the raised leg for about a minute. As you lengthen your right leg, press your first metatarsal against the strap, and firm the inner corner of your right heel. Broaden the balls of your right foot by widening the neck of the little toe away from the ball of the big toe. Then lengthen your left leg against the floor, and firm the inner corner of your left heel. To come out of the pose, bend your right leg, release the strap, and repeat to the other side.

Practice Notes. If you are flexible enough to practice Side-Lying Toe-Holding Pose without a strap, bend your right leg and take hold of your big toe with the second and third fingers of your right hand. Do not pull the big toe forward with your hand. Instead, strengthen the neck of the big toe by firming it against your fingers.

RECLINING POSE

Relaxation Pose

SAVASANA

▼ ▼ ▼ ▼ ▼ ▼ ▼ ▼ ▼ ▼ ▼ ▼

relaxes the legs, ankles, and feet ▪ quiets the breath

Props: 1 nonskid mat ▪ 1 bolster or blanket

Optional Props: 1 or 2 blankets

Relaxation Pose is practiced here with the ankles supported (Figure 35).

Place a bolster or rolled blanket crosswise at the far end of your nonskid mat. Lie on your back with your legs extended, and rest your outer anklebones on the bolster with your feet several inches apart, so that your ankle joints are in line with your hip joints. Relax your legs, ankles, and feet.

If you feel any discomfort or strain in your neck or shoulders, place a folded blanket under your head and neck. Then relax your shoulder blades, and extend your arms away from the sides of your rib cage. Close your eyes gently, and lengthen from the base of your skull to the crown of your head. Relax the skin of your face. Remain in

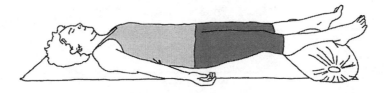

35. RELAXATION POSE, WITH ANKLES SUPPORTED

Relaxation Pose with the ankles supported for 3 to 10 minutes. To come out of the pose, bend your knees and turn onto your side before sitting up.

Practice Notes. If your knees hyperextend in Relaxation Pose with the ankles supported, place another rolled or folded blanket under your knees as well.

Part 3

▼ ▼ ▼ ▼ ▼ ▼ ▼ ▼ ▼ ▼ ▼

Practice Sequences

FAQ

Here are answers to questions often asked by students.

Under what circumstances should I consult my doctor before practicing yoga?

You should consult your doctor before starting a yoga practice if you are taking medication for a chronic health condition, if you suffer from chronic pain, or if you have any apprehension because of your age or physical ability.

Do I need to let my yoga teacher know about my health issues?

If you have a chronic health condition or suffer from chronic pain or injury, you should tell your yoga teacher about it before attending your first class. If you feel uncomfortable about sharing this information in front of others, call or email your teacher in advance of the class. You can also remind the teacher to keep your health concerns confidential, if this is important to you. A well-trained teacher will respect your need for privacy whether you specifically ask for it or not.

How can I begin practicing yoga if I am pregnant?

Find a special class in yoga for pregnancy, if you can. Otherwise you can join a general class, but contact the teacher first to determine whether the class is an appropriate level for you. Be sure to tell the teacher what trimester you are in and if you have a history of miscarriages.

How often should I attend a yoga class?

Most people attend a class once a week, while others attend two or three times a week. You will benefit more from your weekly class if you also practice at home. Start with a 20-to-30-minute yoga session at home once or twice a week, and build from there. Practice the poses you learn in class.

I'm concerned that if I practice on my own, reading from the book, I might not be doing the pose the right way and may injure myself. What do you recommend?

It is unlikely that you will injure yourself if you practice slowly and carefully, with proper attention to alignment. If the pose feels good, it probably is good. If you feel acute discomfort, such as pain in your knees or lower back, come out of the pose immediately and read the instructions once again. Try one of the optional props to see if that helps. If it doesn't help, skip the pose for now and seek advice from an experienced teacher.

Can I practice when I am feeling ill?

Do not continue to practice if you feel feverish, dizzy, nauseous, or breathless.

Is it okay to eat before practicing?

It is best to practice yoga on an empty stomach. A light snack such as a piece of fruit or a piece of toast at least an hour before your practice session begins, or a light meal at least two hours before, is usually okay.

What should I wear to practice yoga?

Wear clothing that does not restrict your movement, such as a t-shirt and shorts or leggings. Avoid tight jeans. If you are practicing at home, it's okay to wear loose-fitting pants, but when attending a class, wear something that allows your teacher to see your knees.

Can I wear my shoes to practice yoga?

We usually practice yoga barefoot so that the soles of our feet become more sensitive to the floor and our feet are not restricted in their movement. However, it may be appropriate for you to wear shoes (1) if you have a fungal infection or rash on your feet that may be contagious; (2) if you need the support of orthotics to maintain your balance in standing poses; or (3) if you are practicing outdoors on a rough surface that might otherwise injure your feet. If you want to wear shoes to class for a particular reason, contact the teacher for permission before attending the class. Have a special pair of shoes that you wear only in the yoga studio so you are not dragging in dirt from outside.

What props do I need for practicing with this book?

1 nonskid mat

2–3 blankets

2 foam, cork, or wooden blocks

2 foam wedges

1 strap with a buckle

2 facecloths

1 bolster

1 wall

Where can I buy props?

The yoga props mentioned in *Yoga for Healthy Feet* can be purchased from Hugger-Mugger Yoga Products, www.huggermugger.com.

PRACTICE SEQUENCE 1: FIND YOUR FEET

The purpose of this sequence is to help you find your feet kinesthetically by developing awareness of your metatarsals, inner and outer arches, and heels. *Most of the poses in this sequence are best practiced without the aid of props, except for a nonskid mat.*

When practicing this sequence, choose one of the three images below (or any other image from this book that resonates with you), and see how it applies to each of the poses in the sequence. You may find that an image works well for you in one pose but not in another. In asymmetrical standing poses, you may find an instruction helpful for the back leg but not for the front leg, or vice versa. If an image doesn't work for you, feel free to alter or adapt it to meet your particular needs. Listen to what your feet are telling you.

- Roll your outer metatarsals toward your outer foot and your first metatarsal toward your inner foot.
- Lift your inner and outer arches evenly.
- Distribute your weight evenly around the circumference of your heel.

1. Mountain Pose
(page 52)
30–60 seconds

2. Chair Pose
(page 61)
30–60 seconds

3. Toe-Holding Pose
(page 56)
30–60 seconds

4. Extended Triangle Pose

(page 58)

30–60 seconds, each side

5. Wide-Leg Standing Forward Bend

(page 70)

30–60 seconds

6. Extended Side-Angle Pose

(page 68)

30–60 seconds, each side

7. Standing Forward Bend

(page 72)

30–60 seconds

8. Half Moon Pose, with Hand on Block

(page 74)

30–60 seconds, each side

9. Warrior I Pose

(page 77)

30–60 seconds, each side

10. Downward-Facing Dog Pose, with Heels Supported

(page 50)

30–60 seconds

11. Relaxation Pose

(page 101)

3–7 minutes

Practice Sequence 2: Strengthen Your Toes

This sequence is intended to strengthen the necks of your toes with the aid of a wedge or other support placed under your toes. The sequence is recommended especially if you have curled or hammertoes or toes that have been weakened by numbness or neuropathy, but it is beneficial for everyone.

The use of a wedge under the toes is described in Chair Pose (page 61) and Warrior Pose II (page 63). Place the wedge under your foot so that the balls of the foot are on your mat and the necks of your toes are supported by the thin edge of the wedge. In asymmetrical poses, the wedge can be turned at an angle to the frontal plane of the foot. (If you do not have a foam wedge, try using a mat folded in half to support the toes. A wooden wedge generally lifts the toes too much.)

Use the pressure of your toes against the wedge to widen the balls of your feet and lengthen your toes. Let the neck of your little toe move away from the ball of your big toe. The wedge can be used in other standing poses, as indicated below.

1. Mountain Pose, with Toes on Wedge
(page 52)
30–60 seconds

2. Chair Pose, with Toes on Wedge
(page 61)
30–60 seconds

3. Extended Triangle Pose, with Toes on Wedge
(page 58)
30–60 seconds, each side

4. Standing Forward Bend, with Toes on Wedge
(page 72)
30–60 seconds

5. Warrior Pose II, with Toes on Wedge
(page 63)
30–60 seconds, each side

6. Wide-Leg Standing Forward Bend, with Toes on Wedges
(page 70)
30–60 seconds

7. Extended Side-Angle Pose, with Toes on Wedge
(page 68)
30–60 seconds, each side

8. Toe-Holding Pose, with Strap on Big Toes
(page 56)
30–60 seconds

9. Half Moon Pose, with Toes on Wedge
(page 74)
30-60 seconds, each side

10. Warrior Pose I, with Toes on Wedge
(page 77)
30–60 seconds, each side

11. Downward-Facing Dog Pose, with Heels Supported
(page 50)
30–60 seconds

12. Side-Lying Toe-Holding Pose, with Strap around Arch
(page 99)
30–60 seconds, each side

13. Relaxation Pose, with Ankles Supported
(page 101)
3–5 minutes

PRACTICE SEQUENCE 3: STABILIZE YOUR FOOT AND ANKLE

This sequence is recommended when you are recovering from a sprained ankle or foot injury. Do not continue to practice any pose that causes pain or discomfort in your foot or ankle.

The use of the wall to stabilize the back foot and strengthen the back leg is described in Extended Triangle Pose (page 58). These instructions can be applied to other standing poses, as indicated below.

1. Downward-Facing Dog Pose, with Heels Supported
(page 50)
30–60 seconds

2. Mountain Pose
(page 52)
30–60 seconds

3. Extended Triangle Pose, with Back Foot at Wall
(page 58)
30–60 seconds, each side

4. Standing Forward Bend, with Feet on Wedges
(page 66)
30–60 seconds

5. Warrior Pose II, with Back Heel at Wall
(page 63)
30–60 seconds, each side

6. Wide-Leg Standing Forward Bend, with Feet on Wedges
(page 70)
30–60 seconds

7. Extended Side-Angle Pose, with Back Foot at Wall
(page 68)
30–60 seconds, each side

8. Standing Forward Bend, with Strap around Arches
(page 72)
30–60 seconds

9. Half Moon Pose, with Back Foot on Wall
(page 74)
30–60 seconds, each side

10. Toe-Holding Pose
(page 56)
30–60 seconds

11. Warrior Pose I, with Back Heel on Wedge
(page 77)
30–60 seconds, each side

12. Downward-Facing Dog Pose, with Heels Supported
(page 50)
30–60 seconds

13. Legs-Up-the-Wall Pose, with Bolster under Pelvis
(page 97)
5–10 minutes

PRACTICE SEQUENCE 4: IMPROVE YOUR BALANCE

This sequence focuses on improving your balance by strengthening your arches and extending the lateral range of motion of your ankle joints.

Review the use of a strap to activate the arches and firm the inner corner of the heels, as described in Reclining Toe-Holding Pose (page 47) and Standing Forward Bend (page 72).

1. Reclining Toe-Holding Pose, with Strap
(page 47)
30–60 seconds, each side

2. Mountain Pose
(page 52)
30–60 seconds

3. Tree Pose, with Knee at Wall
(page 54)
30–60 seconds, each side

4. Extended Triangle Pose
(page 58)
30–60 seconds, each side

5. Standing Forward Bend, with Strap around Arches
(page 72)
30–60 seconds

6. Warrior Pose II
(page 63)
30–60 seconds, each side

7. Wide-Leg Standing Forward Bend, with Feet on Wedges
(page 70)
30–60 seconds

8. Extended Side-Angle Pose, with Inner Foot on Wedge
(page 68)
30–60 seconds, each side

9. Standing Forward Bend, with Feet on Wedges
(page 66)
30–60 seconds

10. Half Moon Pose, with Hand on Block
(page 74)
30–60 seconds, each side

11. Staff Pose, with Strap around Arches
(page 86)
30–60 seconds

12. Head-of-the-Knee Pose, with Ankle Supported
(page 88)
30–60 seconds, each side

13. Bound Angle Pose, with Wedge between Feet
(page 91)
30–60 seconds

14. Relaxation Pose, with Ankles Supported
(page 101)
3–7 minutes

PRACTICE SEQUENCE 5: RELIEVE YOUR OVERSTRESSED ANKLES

This sequence focuses on relieving overstressed ankles and relaxing the bones at the top of the foot. When the ankle joint is forced beyond its normal range of motion, causing pain, discomfort, or cramps, using a support under the ankle can provide relief by restoring the joint to a more neutral position. Take time to adjust the size, shape, and placement of each prop so that you create maximum space and ease in the joint.

This sequence is recommended for those with high arches and others who suffer from foot cramps. For those who want to include Lotus-type poses in their practice, this sequence will help you avoid sickling your foot and overstressing your ankle.

1. Downward-Facing Dog Pose, with Heels Supported
(page 50)
30–60 seconds, each side

2. Simple Seated Twist II, with Inner Foot Supported
(page 81)
30–60 seconds, each side

3. Hero Pose, with Ankles Supported
(page 84)
30–60 seconds

4. Camel Pose, with Feet on Wedge
(page 79)
30–60 seconds

5. Staff Pose, with Strap around Arches
(page 86)
30–60 seconds

6. Bound Angle Pose, with Wedge between Feet
(page 91)
30–60 seconds

7. Head-of-the-Knee Pose, with Ankle Supported
(page 88)
30–60 seconds, each side

9. Half Lotus Staff Pose, with Ankle Supported
(page 93)
30–60 seconds, each side

10. Perfect Pose, with Shinbone Supported
(page 95)
2 minutes, each side

11. Legs-Up-the-Wall Pose, with Bolster under Pelvis
(page 97)
3–7 minutes

12. Relaxation Pose, with Ankles Supported
(page 101)
3 minutes

About the Author

▼ ▼ ▼ ▼ ▼ ▼ ▼ ▼ ▼ ▼ ▼

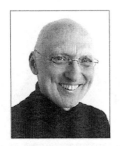

DONALD MOYER, copublisher at Rodmell Press, has been practicing yoga since 1971 and began teaching in 1974. He studied extensively with B.K.S. Iyengar from 1976 to 1987 and remains inspired by his work. In 1978, he founded The Yoga Room in Berkeley, CA. Donald wrote the "Asana" column for *Yoga Journal* in 1987, 1989, and 1992. His columns were pioneering, and his books, *Yoga: Awakening the Inner Body* (2006) and *Yoga for Healthy Feet* (2016), continue to break new ground.

About the Model

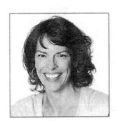

ADA LUSARDI is a graduate and faculty member of The Yoga Room's Advanced Studies Program, in Berkeley, CA. She has been a student of Donald Moyer since 2000. A self-professed anatomy geek, Ada is known for her clear and precise instructions, intelligent sequencing, and skillful hands-on adjustments. She teaches with warmth and humor to students of all ages and abilities. For more information, visit AdaYoga@wordpress.com.

From the Publisher

▼ ▼ ▼ ▼ ▼ ▼ ▼ ▼ ▼ ▼ ▼

SHAMBHALA PUBLICATIONS is pleased to publish the Rodmell Press collection of books on yoga, Buddhism, and aikido. As was the aspiration of the founders of Rodmell Press, it is our hope that these books will help individuals develop a more skillful practice—one that brings peace to their daily lives and to the Earth.

To learn more, please visit www.shambhala.com.

A

Achilles tendon
  illustrated, 42
  lengthening, 39–40
  poses for, 50, 61
Adho Mukha Svanasana. See Downward-Facing
  Dog Pose
aligning
  in asymmetrical standing poses, 24, 26–27
  big toes, 56
  feet, 24–27, 52
  legs with feet, 86
  legs with pelvis, 68
  Mountain Pose for, 17, 27
  in symmetrical standing poses, 24, 25
Anantasana (Side-Lying Toe-Holding Pose),
  99–100, 111
angle of divergence for bunions, 29–30
ankle joint
  of bent leg, pose releasing pressure on, 88
  dorsiflexion, 39–40, 44
  extending range of motion, 42
  outer, pose relieving strain on, 70
  overstressed, practice sequence for relieving,
    116–117
  plantar flexion, 43
  pose balancing inner and outer, 70
  pose draining excess fluid from, 97
  pose enhancing lateral range of motion, 66
  pose increasing flexibility, 61
  pose relaxing, 101
  pose taking pressure off, 77, 79
  poses creating space in, 50, 93
  poses relieving discomfort, 84, 95
  practice sequence for stabilizing, 112–113
  pronation, 42–43
  stiff, pose for, 84

  supination, 43
  unstable, pose for, 66
arches. *See also* inner and outer arches
  collapse in Downward-Facing Dog Pose,
    34–35
  fallen, 34–35, 47, 50
  foot cramping, 40–41, 79, 84
  high, 33, 79, 84
  low, 33–34, 47
  pose activating, 72
  strengthening, 33–34, 47, 86, 91, 99
  weak, poses for, 66, 72
Ardha Chandrasana. See Half Moon Pose
Ardha Padma Dandasana (Half Lotus Staff Pose),
  93–94, 117
asymmetrical standing poses, 24, 26–27, 32

B

back and front foot, 17, 18–19
back bend (Camel Pose), 79–80
back leg, pose stabilizing, 58
Baddha Konasana. See Bound Angle Pose
balance
  in asymmetrical standing poses, 32
  Mountain Pose for, 17
  poses improving, 43, 54, 58, 66
  practice sequence for improving, 114–115
balancing
  front and back foot, 18–19
  inner and outer arches, 32, 40
  top and bottom foot, 18
  widening and lengthening feet, 20
balls of the feet, pose broadening, 52
Bharadvajasana II. See Simple Seated Twist II
big toes
  bunions, 29–32, 56
  circumference of, 25

inner corner of ball of, 31, 34
pose strengthening and aligning, 56
spreading weight evenly around the ball,
    31–32
blood pressure, pose lowering, 97
books, learning yoga from, 9–13, 106
bottom and top foot, 17, 18
Bound Angle Pose (*Baddha Konasana*), 91–92
    inner corner of ball of big toe in, 31
    in practice sequences, 115, 117
    sickling the foot in, 43
breath, pose quieting, 101
bunions, 29–32, 56

C
calcaneus, 37. *See also* heels
calf, outer, strain or burning in, 70
Camel Pose (*Ustrasana*), 40, 79–80, 116
Chair Pose (*Utkatasana*), 61–62
    aligning feet in, 24, 25
    dorsiflexion in, 39–40, 44
    inner corner of ball of big toe in, 31
    in practice sequences, 108, 110
circumference of ball of big toe, 25
circumference of heels, 25, 38
classes, 105–106
claw toes, 28
clothing for yoga practice, 106
conditions
    ankle discomfort, 84, 95
    ankle joint pressure, 77, 79
    bunions, 29–32, 56
    claw toes, 28
    curled toes, 61, 63
    excess fluid in feet, ankles, and legs, 97
    fallen arches, 34–35, 47, 50
    foot cramping, 40–41, 79, 84
    foot discomfort, 84
    foot, pose for recovering from, 58
    groin muscles tight or injured, 68
    hammer toes, 28, 61, 63
    heels not reaching the floor, 37, 50
    high arches, 33, 79, 84
    high blood pressure, 97
    knee hyperextension, 61, 74
    knee pain, 84

knee pressure, 93
knee strain, 81
low arches, 33–34, 47
mallet toes, 27, 28
outer ankle strain, 70
outer calf strain or burning, 70
plantar fasciitis, 38–40, 50, 61
practice during illness, 106
sprained ankle, 41, 58, 70
stiff ankles, 84
tension, 97
unstable ankles, 66
weak arches, 66, 72
cuboid, 23, 36, 37
cuneiform bones, 23
curled toes
    claw toes, 28
    hammer toes, 28
    mallet toes, 27, 28
    poses for, 61, 63

D
Dandasana. See Staff Pose
doctor, consulting, 12–13, 105
dorsiflexion, 39–40, 44
Downward-Facing Dog Pose (*Adho Mukha
    Svanasana*), 50–51
    aligning feet in, 24, 25
    arch collapse in, 34–35
    fallen arches and, 35
    in practice sequences, 109, 111, 112,
        113, 116

E
eating before practice, 106
energy, pose restoring, 97
Extended Side-Angle Pose (*Utthita
    Parsvakonasana*), 68–69
    aligning feet in, 24, 26–27
    in practice sequences, 109, 111, 113, 115
Extended Triangle Pose (*Utthita Trikonasana*),
    58–60
    aligning feet in, 24, 26–27
    balancing feet in, 33
    high arches and, 33
    inner and outer arches in, 32

in practice sequences, 109, 110, 112, 114
sprained ankle and, 41

F
fallen arches, 34–35, 47, 50
FAQ, 105–107
feet. *See also* inner and outer foot; toes
   aligning, 24–27
   developing awareness of, 9
   front and back foot, 17, 18–19
   functions of, 9
   planes of, 17
   pose aligning with legs, 86
   pose draining excess fluid from, 97
   poses relaxing, 93, 101
   practice sequence for awareness of, 108–109
   practice sequence for stabilizing, 112–113
   shape of, 19–22
   shoes and loss of awareness of, 9
   top and bottom foot, 17, 18
   widening and lengthening, 20
Find Your Feet practice sequence, 12,
      108–109
first metatarsal, 23–24
foot cramping, 40–41, 79, 84
foot discomfort, pose relieving, 84
forward bends
   Head-of-the-Knee Pose, 88
   Standing Forward Bend, 66
   Wide-Leg Standing Forward Bend, 70
front and back foot, 17, 18–19
front foot, pose strengthening, 74

G
groin muscles, poses for, 68, 88

H
Half Lotus Staff Pose (*Ardha Padma
      Dandasana*), 93–94, 117
Half Moon Pose (*Ardha Chandrasana*),
      74–76
   aligning feet in, 24, 26–27
   in practice sequences, 109, 111, 113, 115
   Standing Forward Bend as preparation for,
      66–67
hammer toes, 28, 61, 63

Head-of-the-Knee Pose (*Janu Sirsasana*), 88–90
   avoiding dorsiflexion in, 44
   inner corner of ball of big toe in, 31
   in practice sequences, 115, 117
   protecting the knee in, 35
   sickling the foot in, 43
heels
   broadening vs. digging in, 37
   circumference of, 25, 38
   of extended leg, pose supporting, 77
   inner corner of, 34, 38, 72
   not reaching the floor, 37
   not reaching the floor, pose for, 50
   preserving the cushion of, 37
Hero Pose (*Virasana*), 84–85
   foot cramping in, 40, 41
   high arches and, 33
   plantar flexion in, 43
   in practice sequence, 116
high arches, 33, 79, 84
hip joints
   outer, pose releasing, 93
   pose allowing relaxation, 91
   pose opening, 99
   pose releasing, 79
   poses creating space in, 70, 81

I
illness. *See* conditions
Improve Your Balance practice sequence,
      114–115
injuries. *See* conditions
inner and outer ankle joints, pose for, 70
inner and outer arches
   about, 32
   balancing, 40, 52, 74
   illustrated, 34, 36, 37
inner and outer foot
   illustrated, 17
   pose releasing pressure on outer foot, 88
   pose strengthening inner foot, 68
   poses balancing, 47, 81
   as saggital plane, 17
   standing on, 18
inner corner of ball of big toe, 34
inner corner of heel, 34, 38, 72

inverted poses. *See also specific ones*
    Downward-Facing Dog Pose, 50–51
    Legs-Up-the-Wall Pose, 97–98

J
Janu Sirsasana. See Head-of-the-Knee Pose

K
knee
    inner, pose strengthening, 77
    pose countering hyperextension, 61
    pose for avoiding hyperextension, 74
    pose reducing strain on, 81
    pose releasing, 88
    pose relieving pain, 84
    pose taking pressure off, 93
    sitting pose allowing descent of, 91

L
legs
    back, pose stabilizing, 58
    bent, releasing pressure on ankle of, 88
    bent, softening groin muscles of, 88
    extended, pose supporting heel of, 77
    pose aligning with feet, 86
    pose aligning with pelvis, 68
    pose draining excess fluid from, 97
    pose relaxing, 101
Legs-Up-the-Wall Pose (*Viparita Karani*), 97–98,
    113, 117
lengthening
    Achilles tendons, 39–40, 61
    neck, 99
    short and wide feet, 20
    toes, 61, 63
long and narrow feet, 19, 20, 21
Lotus-type poses, preparing for, 88, 93
low arches, 33–34, 47

M
mallet toes, 27, 28
metatarsals, 23–24, 52
Mountain Pose (*Tadasana*), 52–53
    aligning feet in, 24, 25
    aligning toes in, 27

feet together or apart in, 19
importance of, 17
inner and outer arches in, 32
in practice sequences, 108, 110, 112, 114
preserving the cushion of the heels, 38
shape of feet viewed in, 19–22
with Toes on Wedge, 53

N
navicular, 23, 34, 35, 36, 37
neck, pose lengthening, 99

O
outer and inner ankle joints, pose for, 70
outer arch. *See* inner and outer arches
outer foot. *See* inner and outer foot
outer metatarsals, 24

P
Padangusthasana. See Toe-Holding Pose
pelvis, pose aligning with legs, 68
Perfect Pose (*Siddhasana*), 95–96, 117
planes of the feet, 17
plantar fasciitis, 38–40, 50, 61
plantar flexion, 43
Practice Notes for poses, about, 11
practice sequences
    Find Your Feet, 12, 108–109
    Improve Your Balance, 114–115
    Relieve Your Overstressed Ankles, 116–117
    Stabilize Your Foot and Ankle, 33, 41, 112–113
    Strengthen Your Toes, 110–111
    time required for, 12
    using, 11–12
Prasarita Padottanasana. See Wide-Leg Standing
    Forward Bend
pregnancy, yoga practice during, 105
problems. *See* conditions
pronation, 42–43
props, 11, 107

R
reclining poses. *See also specific ones*
    Reclining Toe-Holding Pose, 47–49
    Relaxation Pose, 101–102
    Side-Lying Toe-Holding Pose, 99–100

Reclining Toe-Holding Pose (*Supta Padangusthasana*), 47–49
  activating inner corner of heel in, 38
  dorsiflexion work in, 39
  with Leg to Side, 48–49
  with Leg Up, 48
  plantar flexion in, 43
  in practice sequence, 114
Relaxation Pose (*Savasana*), 101–102
  in practice sequences, 109, 111, 115, 117
Relieve Your Overstressed Ankles practice sequence, 116–117

S
Savasana (Relaxation Pose), 101–102
  in practice sequences, 109, 111, 115, 117
second metatarsal, 23, 24, 37
shape of feet, 19–22
shoes, 9, 39, 106–107
short and wide feet, 20, 22
shoulders, pose relaxing, 99
sickling the foot, avoiding, 43
Siddhasana (Perfect Pose), 95–96, 117
Side-Lying Toe-Holding Pose (*Anantasana*), 99–100, 111
Simple Seated Twist II (*Bharadvajasana II*), 81–83
  in practice sequence, 116
  protecting the knee in, 35
  sickling the foot in, 43
sitting poses. *See also specific ones*
  Bound Angle Pose, 91–92
  Half Lotus Staff Pose, 93–94
  Hero Pose, 84–85
  Perfect Pose, 95–96
  Staff Pose, 86–87
sprained ankle, 41, 58, 70
Stabilize Your Foot and Ankle practice sequence, 33, 41, 112–113
Staff Pose (*Dandasana*), 86–87
  activating inner corner of heel in, 38
  avoiding dorsiflexion in, 44
  in practice sequences, 115, 116
Standing Forward Bend (*Uttanasana*)
  activating inner corner of heel in, 38
  aligning feet in, 24, 25

  balance improved by, 43
  inner corner of ball of big toe in, 31
  in practice sequences, 109, 110, 112, 113, 114, 115
  sickling the foot and, 43
  with strap, 72–73
  on wedges, 66–67
standing poses. *See also specific ones*
  asymmetrical, 24, 26–27
  barefoot, as revitalizing, 9
  Chair Pose, 61–62
  Extended Side-Angle Pose, 68–69
  Extended Triangle Pose, 58–60
  Half Moon Pose, 74–76
  heel not reaching the floor in, 37
  high arches and, 33
  learning from, 10
  Mountain Pose, 52–53
  Standing Forward Bend, 66–67, 70–71
  symmetrical, 24, 25
  Toe-Holding Pose, 56–57
  Tree Pose, 54–55
  Warrior Pose I, 77–78
  Warrior Pose II, 63–65
  Wide-Leg Standing Forward Bend, 70–71
Strengthen Your Toes practice sequence, 110–111
strengthening
  arches, 33–34, 47, 86, 91, 99
  big toes, 56
  front foot, 74
  inner corner of ball of big toe, 31
  inner corner of heel, 72
  inner foot, 68
  inner knee, 77
  inner thighs, 54
  metatarsals, 52
  toes, 61, 63, 110–111
supination, 43
Supta Padangusthasana. See Reclining Toe-Holding Pose
symmetrical standing poses, 24, 25, 32

T
Tadasana. See Mountain Pose
tarsals, 23, 35–37

tension, pose reducing, 97
thighs, pose strengthening inner, 54
Toe-Holding Pose (*Padangusthasana*), 56–57
  aligning feet in, 24, 25
  in practice sequences, 108, 111, 113
toes, 27–29
  aligning in Mountain pose, 27
  claw, 28
  curled, 61, 63
  hammer, 28, 61, 63
  lengthening, 61, 63
  mallet, 27, 28
  straightening, exercise for, 28–29
  strengthening, 61, 63, 110–111
top and bottom foot, 17, 18
Tree Pose (*Vrksasana*), 54–55, 66, 114
twisting pose (Simple Seated Twist II), 81–83

U
using this book, 9–13
Ustrasana (Camel Pose), 40, 79–80, 116
Utkatasana. See Chair Pose
Uttanasana. See Standing Forward Bend
Utthita Parsvakonasana. See Extended
    Side-Angle Pose
Utthita Trikonasana. See Extended Triangle Pose

V
Viparita Karani (Legs-Up-the-Wall Pose),
    97–98, 113, 117
Virabhadrasana I (Warrior Pose I).
    See Warrior Pose I

Virabhadrasana II (Warrior Pose II).
    See Warrior Pose II
Virasana. See Hero Pose
Vrksasana (Tree Pose), 54–55, 66, 114

W
Warrior Pose I (*Virabhadrasana I*)
  heel not reaching the floor in, 37
  in practice sequences, 109, 111, 113
Warrior Pose II (*Virabhadrasana II*), 63–65
  aligning feet in, 24, 26–27
  in practice sequences, 111, 112, 114
Wide-Leg Standing Forward Bend (*Prasarita
    Padottanasana*), 70–71
  aligning feet in, 24, 25
  in practice sequences, 109, 111, 112, 115
  sickling the foot in, 43
widening long and narrow feet, 20

Y
yoga classes, 105–106
yoga practice
  beginning during pregnancy, 105
  clothing for, 106
  consulting doctor before, 12–13, 105
  eating before, 106
  general cautions for, 12–13
  during illness, 106
  learning from a book, 9–13, 106
  props for, 107
  using the poses in part 2, 10–11
  wearing shoes for, 106–107

Printed in the United States
by Baker & Taylor Publisher Services